Adrenal Fatigue

Lukas
McGregor

Adrenal Fatigue

An epidemic known only
to your contemporaries...
and how to deal with it

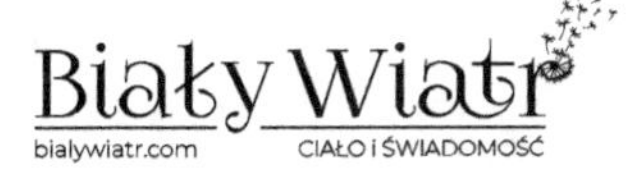

 All medical information given in this publication is for educational purposes only. It is not the intention of the author for it to be used for diagnostic or therapeutic purposes. The information presented cannot replace professional diagnosis and treatment. Prior to making any decisions regarding your health, medical consultation is advised. Neither the author nor the publisher is liable for any type of damages resulting from the use of the knowledge contained herein.

Table of Contents

Introduction

Undoubtedly, we live in times full of challenges. Our prehistoric ancestors would not be capable of imagining a world in which clean water is a luxury, meat that comes from animals living in unnatural conditions and are fed with harmful chemicals, and drinks and meals that are purchased in cardboard packaging. It would surely be difficult for them to understand the phenomenon of GMO, air pollution caused by factory emissions or automobile exhaust, the qualitative depletion of soils caused by fertilizers, heavy metal poisoning, and excessive exposure to electromagnetic radiation or light twenty four hours a day, in the form of electricity. They would not be able to perceive life in the constant hurry that affects modern man as well as the stress associated with the daily deadlock of traffic jams, struggling with despised bosses, unemployment, financial difficulties or the challenges connected with being a parent, problems in relationships, or the illnesses of our loved ones. The World Health Organization (WHO) estimates that by the year 2020 ailments and illnesses due to stress will be the second leading cause of human illness worldwide.

Although each of us reacts in a slightly different way to stressful situations, the body generally exhibits a certain characteristic response to this type of stimulation. It is a mechanism which has evolved over millions of years in the course of evolution, and which can briefly be described as a fight or flight reaction.

This reaction has been biologically programmed within us and has been operating from the time when primitive humans who on their way encountered a mammoth, a tiger, or another predator and had to react with one of the three behaviors – fight, flee, or remain motionless. Stress in the Palaeolithic Age was, as a rule, very intense, but it lasted a short time, and occurred relatively rarely. Today, it is completely different. As for our ancestors, after struggling with difficult situations they had time to regenerate as well as prepare for the next confrontation with demanding living conditions or wildlife. Modern man is exposed to stressful stimuli that often disappear quickly or there is just too much. Furthermore, these stimuli very often possess a typically mental nature. Each time we come into contact with some complication or obstacle, such as problems at work, educational difficulties, a personal illness, or the illness of someone close to us, our body reacts the same as if there were a dangerous predator in our way, and thus a life-threatening situation appears. We live under the pressure of time, obligations, deadlines with a multi-point list of daily issues to be dealt with, and bombarded with information and advertising. The enormous amount of factors from morning till evening causes constant overstimulation. Television and internet alone provide as much stimuli per week as our Paleolithic ancestors had throughout their whole lives. Unfortunately, nature has provided us with bodies and mechanisms which permit us to deal with only one roaring mammoth or lion at a time, and not a whole jungle of stimuli. The brain of modern man is too overloaded to deal with sorting out all of the daily information and events which arise, and certainly not that which a fresh pair of eyes might determine what to do with them all.

All the more so that our reaction to fight or flight does not understand the concept of distance. Often, even when we read or watch information concerning wars, illnesses, terrorist attacks or catastrophes happening elsewhere in the world, or we hear worrisome information about economics or politics, our biology reacts more quickly than a thinking brain, which is aware that everything is happening in another time or place. The impetus of danger, heightened by unsettling thoughts and emotions put a whole cascade of physical, neurological and hormonal processes in motion. It causes tension, anxiety, internal cramps, and a feeling of insecurity. The pulse quickens and a larger amount of blood is pumped into the muscles making them ready for action; often completely unnecessarily. First of all, because we simply don't have much influence on many things; and secondly, due to the amount of stimuli, our reaction to the stress is disproportionate to the potential threat. Unfortunately, if the body and brain remain in a state of chronic and permanent stress, it shifts onto the functioning of all internal systems and various illnesses appear.

One of the ailments of the modern world outright increasing in epidemic proportions is hypoadrenia, or so-called adrenal fatigue. Probably most of us – if not everyone – have weakened adrenal glands, as evidenced by many of the somatic symptoms that we experience every day. Dr. Michael Lam, a medical authority in this field, claims that probably several times throughout our lifespan each of us suffers, or has suffered, as a result of a greater impairment of these glands. This may be caused by a change in residence, demanding exams during studies, an excess of responsibilities at work, financial difficulties, losing one's job or unemployment, or demands connected with the parenting of a small child or support for a disabled or ill member of the family.

Such situations and life turbulence do not remain indifferent to the state of our health and well-being. It results in a distortion to the endocrine system and various physical symptoms. Good if the stress factor subsides or eases ... then, usually without specific remedial measures and after some time, the body regains its equilibrium itself. Worse, if the stressors overlap themselves or last for a long time. Then, the adaptive mechanisms break down and we need specific help. Knowledge is all the more valuable in how to support the functioning of the adrenal glands (widely used in all types of stress response) so that they can again function optimally.

The primary purpose of this study is the concise characteristics of weakening adrenal glands in the context of the topic of stress which affects modern man, as well as the fact that western medicine does not recognize this ailment as a disease classification and therefore officially does not treat it. The author of this manuscript is depending on drawing the attention of doctors and ordinary people who are interested in state of their own health, and who would like to take appropriate measures on their own.

FOREWORD TO THE SECOND EDITION

When I wrote this study eight years ago, I didn't expect it to be received so warmly. I endeavoured to compile the necessary and practical essence of knowledge on the subject of the adrenal gland, and that is precisely what has been appreciated. I am very grateful for that!

However, time does not stand still, just like discoveries in various fields. And although, as I observe, little has changed in terms of the approach to adrenal fatigue (the medical community still does not take this issue seriously), and social awareness remains low, I deemed it worthwhile to update and supplement some information that appeared in the first edition. Especially when you consider that the overall level of stress in the population has increased, not decreased. As individuals, we are facing more and more challenges that are having an impact on our health and ability to function.

In light of the above, this second edition of Adrenal Fatigue includes additional suggestions for stress reduction, an updated approach to diet, and new suggestions for supplementation to strengthen weakened adrenal glands and the nervous system.

STRESS AND ITS EFFECT ON THE BODY

To better understand the risk associated with weakened adrenal glands, it is initially worth observing the very nature of stress itself, its biochemical mechanisms, as well as the effects it has on the human body. Obviously, it is not only stress that weakens the adrenal glands – there are several other causes that we will discuss later. Nevertheless, it is in fact its chronic character that seems to be the primary cause of this condition. Stress can impact many different levels – physiological, psychological, and social, which all react to one other.

A bit of history

The first scientific study on stress is owed to Dr. Walter Bradford Cannon (1871-1945), a graduate of Harvard University who, already in his youth, was drawn to the science behind emotion and the influence of environmental factors on the human body. He noted, among other things, that when the animals participating in his experiments became frightened or disturbed, the normal peristaltic movements in their stomach suddenly ceased. After completing his medical studies, Cannon became the chairman of the Physiology Department at Harvard and began comprehensive research into the physiology of emotion – becoming the first recognized researcher in this field. He pointed out, among other things, that when an animal is extremely agitated, its nervous system mobilizes the "fight or flight" reaction. In the words of Cannon – the sympatoadrenal system produces changes in blood supply, blood sugar availability, as well as coagulation in the face of the "sudden appearance of a stressor."

In 1915, he summarized his work in the groundbreaking book, "Bodily Changes in Pain, Hunger, Fear and Rage." In 1917, his knowledge in the field of physiology assisted in the development of life-saving resuscitation procedures on the battlefield, particularly in the rapid replenishment of fluids lost from blood flow. After the war, Cannon moved on from the scientific aspect of physiology to its clinical application, becoming a major authority in the emergence of a new field of psychosomatic medicine.

Although Walter Cannon is considered a precursor to stress and emotion research and their relationship to health, Hans Hugo Seyle (1907-1982), a brilliant scientist, physiopathologist, and endocrinologist of Hungarian descent, is considered the creator of the very concept of stress.

It is Selye himself who hypothesized that a number of somatic illnesses are the result of one's inability to deal with constant stress. He devoted 50 years of scientific work to researching this phenomenon and its impact on human health, and which has been documented in more than 1,600 articles as well as the first book devoted to stress, The Stress of Life (1956).

He wrote about it in this way:

Enormous stress caused, for instance, by long periods of hunger, fear for one's life, fatigue, or chills can overwhelm or even destroy the body's defense mechanisms. (…) For this reason, some illnesses spread rapidly during periods of war or famine. Since parasites, bacteria, or viruses constantly remain in our environment, yet illnesses are only result when we experience stress – what is the cause of the illness – these external or internal intruders, or stress? In my opinion, both factors are equally responsible for this.

Seyle's interest in the body's physiological response to stress had already begun in 1925 during medical studies. At first, they were individual reactions to illnesses and physical ailments. The curriculum included, among others, observing patients in the early phases of various infectious diseases. The professor noticed that the patients "looked and felt sick, and had digestive problems and depression." He described these symptoms as "unspecified" and useless in attempting to identify the pathogens responsible for it or for genetic factors. However, he disagreed that these symptoms were considered useless only because they were unspecified. He posed the question as to why various illnesses, such as allergies and infections, have similar unspecified symptoms. He also noticed the characteristic biological pattern of the body adapting to external stressors in order to maintain an inner equilibrium. In its attempt to preserve homeostasis, the body uses specific hormones in a fight or flight reaction. Selye discovered that even if the body wants to control or reduce stress, it still has its limitations. This limited ability to adapt to stress is even more noticeable when the body is exposed to the long-term effects of a stressor. Despite being discouraged by his colleagues, he came to discover and isolate the three-phased role of hormones in their response to stress. This created the basis for what was called General Adaptation Syndrome (GAS):

1st stage: Alarm

This is an immediate response to an internal or external stressor – "fight or flight." The body perceives the factor as a threat or danger and releases stress hormones such as adrenaline or cortisol. These hormones allow the body to act in excess of its normal capabilities. For instance, at the moment of injury, the immune system activates an appropriate inflammatory condition with the aim of stopping possible bleeding. The reaction to a stressor is usually quick, specific, and infallible.

2nd stage: Resistance (adaptation)

This appears after the body has decisively responded to the stressor and the level of stress has been reduced or removed. The body's protection weakens as it needs to transfer energy to damaged tissues or weakened systems. Although the body has moved onto the second GAS phase, it remains alert, especially when the stressors have not subsided and the body still needs to fight them. If the stressful situation is prolonged, physiological processes attempt to adapt us to it, resulting in the body instinctively beginning to release more stress hormones to help cope with the situation.

3rd stage: Exhaustion

With long-term stressors (depending on individual predisposition, for several days to several weeks or even months), the body begins to lose the ability to overcome the stressor and reduce its harmful effect – adaptive energy succumbs to exhaustion. This leads to "burnout" or "stress overload," creating an environment in which a person is exposed to health problems. At this stage, specific illnesses or somatic symptoms may occur. The immune system begins, for example, to permanently maintain a state of inflammation, which will lead to stress-related digestive, skin, or circulatory ailments, while simultaneously impairing the ability to combat viral or bacterial infections.

Of course, not every type of stress is bad. So-called acute stress lasts relatively briefly and is generally beneficial. Stress hormones can have a motivating affect on the body, increase mental acuity and increase enthusiasm. It's only long-term stress that has negative consequences. This is due to the fact that our cells are constantly subjected to removing the toxic metabolic products associated with elevated stress hormones being released into the bloodstream.

Seyle called the unhealthy, destructive type of stress *distress*; while the reinforcing, motivating stress – *eustress*.

The next part of stress research was developed by Thomas Holmes and Richard Rahe, psychiatrists at the University of Washington in Seattle (their research was published in 1967). Their alternative concept is based on the notion of stress connected to specific situations. Scholars have developed a scale of 43 life events which are ranked according to how great an adaptation and effort the body requires of each of them. Pursuant to this order, each situation was assigned a certain point value. This is how the renowned Social Readjustment Rating Scale (SRRS) came to be.

This questionnaire was recommended to people brought to a hospital emergency department, as well as to those accompanying them. It turned out that the sick people experienced many more stressful events in the course of the year preceding their illness than those accompanying them. The statistical relationship between stressors and illness has been proven.

Here are certain stressors expressed in points (out of 100 points)

- Death of a spouse (100)
- Divorce (75)
- Marriage (50)
- Pregnancy (40)
- Gaining a new family member (39)
- Large mortgage on a home (32)

Certain stressors connected with employment:
- Dismissal (47)
- Retirement (45)
- Business readjustment (39)
- A change of one's position at work (36)
- A change in the range of responsibilities (29)
- A spouse starts or stops work (26)
- Trouble with the boss (23)
- A change in working hours or conditions of employment (20)

As one can see, not only so-called negative situations are associated with increased susceptibility to stress and its associated effects. Many life changes such as marriage, a promotion, or other personal accomplishments that are usually treated as "happy" events can cause profound life-changing changes which cause stress. In Seyle's terms, they are examples of eustress, meaning "good stress" and whether in the future they will be shown to be positive for us and for our health depends on our adaptability. If we easily adapt – eustress will be relatively innocent and harmless. It will not threaten to overpower the body's defense systems. However, if adaptation is going to be defiant, even a positive change in life can turn into harmful stress (or what Seyle called it – distress)

Contemporary scientific literature distinguishes 12 types of stress

EMOTIONAL STRESS / marriage, financial pressure, unemployment /

COGNITIVE STRESS / excessive requirements of yourself and life, expectations from other people, under pressure from media /

SENSORIAL STRESS / persistent noise, chronic pain, excessive physical effort /

METABOLIC STRESS / circulatory problems, blood sugar levels, a disruption of PH in the body /

TOXIC STRESS / water and air pollution, the presence of heavy metals, artificial food additives, cosmetics and cleaning agents, and smog /

IMMUNE SYSTEM STRESS / allergies, food intolerance, complications resulting from an improper diet, autoimmune diseases, heavy metal poisoning, and chronic inflammatory conditions /

ENDOCRINOLOGICAL STRESS / Hormonal imbalance, menopause, insulin resistance, neurotransmitter deficiencies /

INFECTIOUS STRESS / viruses, bacteria, parasites, fungi /

OXIDATIVE STRESS / associated with the veins and arteries; a lack of fresh air, and difficulty breathing while sleeping /

STRUCTURAL STRESS / physical injury, ailments connected with the spine /

ENERGETIC STRESS / electromagnetic radiation; radio waves, microwaves, modulated ultrasounds, X-rays, gamma rays /

TRAUMA RELATED STRESS /the death of a loved one, war, catastrophe, terrorist attack, and memories from the past /

SPIRITUAL STRESS /a lack of a sense of purpose in life, a lack of higher values, feelings and emotions /

STRESS CAUSED BY AN IMPROPER DIET OR LIFESTYLE /lack of sleep, irregular and inadequate meals, and an excess of coffee, sugar, alcohol, cigarettes, and narcotics/

There is no way to completely protect oneself from stress. It is inscribed in the human condition and life on this planet. The body has formed the proper mechanisms that help in dealing with it. As we will show during this elaboration, stress also has its positive sides and it is often not worth getting stressed with stress itself. Nevertheless, any kind of stress – if it is prolonged and is not balanced by appropriate behavior that reduces its effects, can lead to a weakening of the body's defense structures and expose it to physical ailments – among others, adrenal fatigue.

The Biochemistry of Stress

Two biological systems are involved in stress response in the body – the **Sympathetic Nervous System** (SNS), which activates first; and the **Hypothalamic Pituitary Adrenal Axis** (HPAA), which kicks in after a certain time.

The **Sympathetic Nervous System** (a part of the autonomic nervous system), which innervates the internal organs, is responsible for the initial fight or flight reaction. In the first moments after a response to a stressor it stimulates the adrenal gland into releasing catecholamines – adrenaline, noradrenaline and dopamine. They must prepare the body for action. Meanwhile, the bronchi expands, breathing deepens, the liver releases the additional blood glucose essential for efficient muscle work, the pupils dilate, blood vessels narrow, and blood thickens (in preparation for possible injury). The heart starts to beat faster, blood pressure rises, however blood is not distributed evenly to all the organs. Less blood finds its way to the skin or digestive system, as its primary transport is directed to the muscles, the heart, and the brain – the organs that are crucial in fight or flight.

Catecholamines more or less function for an hour before being absorbed by the tissues.

If we still feel the need to remain in a state of increased readiness, the body moves onto the next stage.

The **Hypothalamic-Pituitary-Adrenal System** activates a few (dozen) minutes or even longer from a response to a stressor. The hypothalamus activates the pituitary gland, which secretes corticotropin-releasing hormone (CRH). The frontal lobe of the pituitary gland, under the influence of CRH secretes another hormone – corticotropin (adrenocorticotropic hormone, abbreviated ACTH). Corticotropin is transported to the adrenal cortex, which is the impulse for the secretion of glucocorticoids (including cortisol). Cortisol is intended to provide "fuel" for the body. It increases blood glucose and speeds up the breakdown of fatty acids into ketones. Its task is to rearrange the body so that it is able to keep the mobilization as long as possible – it ensures a constant supply of "fuel" – that is, glucose, to the brain and muscles, stimulates fat cells to accumulate reserves, and increases insulin secretion, which means an increased appetite. Simultaneously, cortisol shuts down those processes that are temporarily less important for survival. It suppresses the effects of the immune system, the digestive system, the tissue restoration system, the reproductive system, and higher brain functions – analyzing, memorizing and learning.

As you can see, the adrenal glands play a very vital role in the basic mechanism of stress response and are present in each of its phases.

How the body reacts

Of course, the whole body will suffer from prolonged stress. This is a result of excess cortisol being released into the bloodstream. When such a situation becomes chronic (we are talking about so-called hypercortisol), the fight or flight reaction is practically never silenced. It comes down to maladjustment of the nervous system and the hormonal system, followed by all the rest. These are the systems and organs that are particularly susceptible to long-term stress:

Brain – Elevated amyloid beta levels in the brain. Plaque characteristic of Alzheimer's Disease arise from its deposits and damage brain tissue. Memory, concentration, and learning ability grow weaker. The hippocampus (a small structure situated in the temporal lobe) possesses many cortisol receptors, thus during long-term stress, when cortisol is continually flooding the body, it may damage it.

Migraines and chronic headaches – under the influence of adrenaline, the muscles are alternately excessively expanding and contracting, and the nervous system is overly excited. As a result of these changes, a headache – first felt in the temples and then spreading to the entire head. The pain is pulsating as if someone were squeezing a band on the head. This ailment may be accompanied by stiffness in the neck and symptoms typical for a migraine: photophobia, hypersensitivity to noise.

Bronchi, lungs – For people suffering from asthma or lung disease, i.e. emphysema, it may be difficult to obtain the oxygen needed to breathe. Some studies show that extreme stress, such as the death of a loved one, for example, can actually trigger asthma attacks, shrinking the airways. Stress can cause rapid breathing or hyperventilation, which leads some people to panic attacks.

Hair – emotional stress and physiological stress (under eating, high fever, and metabolic disorders) can lead to hair thinning or so called alopecia areata.

Circulatory system – under stress, nerves release the neuropeptide Y into the bloodstream, which raises heart rate and blood pressure. It increases the risk of heart attack and stroke. Chronic stress can also raise the overall cholesterol level.

Skin – High cortisol slows the skin's regenerative processes and accelerates the appearance of wrinkles. Blemishes and red spots may appear on the face and neckline. Sometimes urticaria occurs. The symptoms of common acne and rosacea (rosy color, red lumps and pimples, itching and burning skin) are exacerbated.

Anabolic-catabolic balance disorder– cortisol as a catabolic hormone displaces DHEA – an anabolic hormone. There is a reduction in the synthesis of amino acids, which leads to a reduction in muscle mass. A protein deficiency affects not only the general musculature but also other organs such as the heart, bones, or lining of the gastrointestinal tract.

Neurological problems – problems with concentration, permanent anxiety, neurosis, insomnia, and depression. Dizziness, a reduced tolerance to temperature and weather changes, numbness and tingling of the extremities, and excessive sweating are also possible.

Sleep – Frequent waking in the middle of the night between 1am and 3am, most often as a result of a decrease in blood glucose. This can be accompanied by palpitations and a racing heart, nightmares, cold sweats, and severe anxiety.

Immune system and digestion – Long-lasting stress causes the blood to drain from the digestive tract, especially from the intestines, which causes its lining to not be properly regenerated. The composition of the bacterial flora changes, which has an influence on the functioning of both the digestive system and immune system. Acidification increases in the body which causes the amount of beneficial bacteria to decrease (they take part in the production of many vitamins and support the absorption of electrolytes, allowing for proper fermentation), and increase the amount of pathogenic fungi (e.g. candida). It creates an environment conducive to other parasites

Muscles and joints – chronic tense muscles can ache. Tension headaches and migraine headaches are associated with chronic muscle contraction in the area of the arms, neck, and head.

Pancreas – a persistent elevated blood sugar level under the influence of cortisol leads to insulin resistance and is conducive to the development of insulin resistance.

Osteoporosis – an excess of stress hormones disrupts calcium metabolism and stores it in the bones. It however increases excretion of this element through the kidneys. It is conducive to bone degeneration and increases osteoporosis.

Stomach – a narrowing of the blood vessels may damage the gastric mucosa over time.

Fatty tissue – An excess of cortisol results in a decrease in the consumption of glucose as fuel. Due to more glucose in the bloodstream, more insulin is produced by the pancreas which blocks the release of fatty acids from the cells. In this way fatty tissue is deposited around the abdomen. Abdominal obesity is one of the factors contributing to the development of type 2 diabetes.

As we can see, stress exerts various effects on the whole body. High levels of cortisol keep the body in an unnatural state of continual heightened readiness. However, this situation does not last forever. Depending on individual predisposition – for some it is faster, for others it is slower – there is a dramatic decrease in cortisol. It indicates the final phase of an overload of the stress regulation system.

THE ADRENAL GLAND – COMPOSITION, PHYSIOLOGY, AND FUNCTIONS

The adrenal glands, despite being part of the so-called HPA axis (Hypothalamic-Pituitary-Adrenal Gland), are located at a considerable distance from the remaining glands. They are located in the middle of the lower half of the back, just above the kidneys. Hence their name (Latin *ad renes*, English *adrenal*, meaning close to the kidneys). The influence of the adrenal glands on the functioning of the kidneys themselves is very intense, as they release aldosterone which helps the kidneys in absorbing sodium to retain electrolytes and water in the blood.

An interesting fact is that each adrenal gland has a distinctive shape – the right has a triangular shape, while the left resembles a crescent. Their size (approx. 6 cm by 2.5 cm) and their hues (yellowish) are the same.

Adrenal hormones act on all the important physiological processes in the body – they regulate blood sugar levels and have an influence on the consumption of carbohydrates and fats. Their role is also to direct the process of converting fats and proteins into energy.

Three layers can be distinguished in the adrenal gland– the capsule, the cortex, and the medulla.

The **CAPSULE** is a protective layer. It represents a minimal percentage of the mass of the whole organ. It surrounds and protects every adrenal gland. This is an essential function.

The **CORTEX** (approx. 80% of the gland's mass) completely surrounds the medulla hidden in the center and is responsible for the production of 40 different hormones. Its functions are spread over three separate zones. From the outside (i.e. the protective capsule), the medulla is protected by: a) the zona glomerulosa (glomerular layer), (b) the zona fasciculata (fascicular layer), and c) the zona reticularis (reticular layer). Although all are found within the cortex, their tasks are somewhat different. They are:

a) zona glomerulosa (glomerular layer) – The outermost layer of the cortex produces mineralocorticoids (including aldosterone) that regulate sodium and potassium levels in the blood, thus contributing to properly maintaining the water-electrolyte management of the system. Moreover, it regulates blood pressure, the heart, and skeletal muscles, as well as affects the functioning of the circulatory system;

b) Zona fasciculata (fascicular layer) – The central layer of the cortex, mainly managing the level of corticosteroids, which include cortisol and its derivatives.

Cortisol is one of the most important hormones in the body. It controls sleep rhythm and alertness, digestion, blood pressure, feelings of hunger, as well as physical activity, and it also affects carbohydrate management.

Here are some of the other functions of cortisol:

- strengthens the natural immunity and endurance of the body,
- helps to regulate mood and maintain emotional stability,
- is an effective anti-allergic agent, often used in first aid procedures in the event of shock,
- stimulates the liver to convert amino acids into glucose – the main fuel for energy production,
- maintains resistance to stress as a result of infections, physical traumas, emotional traumas, extreme temperatures, etc.,
- determines how much sodium we have in our blood,
- stabilizes the heart and circulation,
- regulates the strength of connective tissues,
- releases fatty acids (from fat cells) and increases their level in the blood,
- suppresses excessive cell proliferation and, as a consequence, cancerous degradation,

– increases blood coagulation by increasing the amount of platelets in the blood, therefore it is extremely useful in the management of bleeding, e.g. in people suffering from hemophilia.

c) zona reticularis (reticular layer) – the innermost layer of the cortex with a steroid composition and masculinizing effect which produces and secretes sex hormones, and physiologically occurs in men and in women in low concentrations (it include DHEA, DHEA-5, as well as androstenedione).

For people with adrenal fatigue, the hormone DHEA is of key importance. It is an indication of the wisdom of the body and that every function of the body has an inverse function. Under normal circumstances, DHEA reverses many of the adverse effects of excessive cortisol and is released when the "danger passes," allowing the body to regenerate. Healthy functioning glands are able to maintain this balance. However, people suffering from weakened adrenal glands usually have lowered levels of DHEA (cortisol produced in chronically elevated amounts inhibits the production of DHEA), so oftentimes an indication of supplementation from the outside appears – especially taking into account the fact that in one way or another it decreases with age.

Here are some other essential functions of DHEA:

- Improves the functioning of the cardiovascular system by lowering the level of LDL ("bad" cholesterol)
- stimulates the formation of bone tissue as well as its reconstruction, which prevents osteoporosis,
- functions as an androgen, assisting the body in developing muscle tissue; reduces fatty tissue,
- Is a precursor of testosterone and estrogen (hormones associated with sexual arousal),
- improves the immune system, increasing resistance to viruses, bacteria, yeasts, parasites, allergies, and tumors,
- Affects the clarity of the mind, sleep, vitality; assists the body in recovering from extreme stress, which is associated with a lack of sleep, excessive exercise, or emotional problems.

The **MEDULLA** (approx . 20% of the mass of the gland) differs from the structural as well as functional cortex and has one essential function; namely, it affects our reaction to fight or flight through neurotransmitters generating an initial response to stress.

Hormones produced by the medulla are:

- adrenaline – takes part in stress response, causes an increase in heart rate, an increase in blood pressure, expands the bronchi, dilates the pupils, increases the

concentration of glucose in the blood by intensifying
the distribution of glycogen in the liver;
- noradrenaline – causes and increase in heart rate, an
  increase in blood pressure through contraction of the
  peripheral vessels, expansion of the coronary vessels,
  an increase in muscle tension, dilated pupils, increases
  the concentration of glucose in the blood by intensifying the distribution of glycogen in the liver;
- dopamine – Increases the strength of heart muscle contractions as well as increases renal blood flow
  through the enlargement of renal vessels;

HYPOADRENIA – CAUSES SYMPTOMS, AND THE PHASES OF FATIGUE

When did it begin...

The first mention of adrenal glands comes from the eighteenth century, when doctors first began to understand the functions of these glands and recognize the dysfunction associated with them. The set of symptoms and the term "adrenal fatigue," however, came much later, only near the end of the twentieth century (in 1998) and was first used by Dr. James Wilson. Previous research focused on the more specific diseases of these organs.

The first of them – Addison's disease – was first recognized by Dr. Thomas Addison, who presented it to the London Medical Association in 1849 as "the state of general anemia in an adult male." Today, Addison's disease is characterized by the progressive inefficiency and degeneration of the adrenal glands. The cause of Addison's disease is not well known, but doctors suspect it is an auto-immune disease. Adrenal gland damage can be caused by tuberculosis, and pituitary or cancerous diseases. Adrenal insufficiency can occur after the withdrawal of a constant intake of steroids. Officially, medicine does not associate Addison's disease with progressive adrenal fatigue resulting from stress.

Another adrenal gland dysfunction treated as a specific disease is so-called Cushing's syndrome (hypercortisolism). Most often, this disease results from the prolonged administration of GKS as an anti-inflammatory drug (e.g. as a result of rheumatoid arthritis) – we then say exogenous (so-called iatrogenic) Cushing syndrome. The remaining cases, caused by excessive adrenal cortisol synthesis, are termed as endogenous (non-iatrogenic) Cushing syndrome – which may be associated to tumors in the adrenal gland itself which produce too much cortisol, or pituitary tumors.

In the late 19th nineteenth century, doctors began using porcine adrenal cells to treat Addison's disease. The first known use of this procedure in 1898 can be attributed to the doctor, Sir William Osler, exactly one hundred years before our contemporary Dr. Wilson renamed subclinical hypoadrenia to adrenal fatigue. Although Osler's first attempts were unsuccessful, adrenal extracts would later become a very popular treatment option, despite eventually being replaced by more inexpensive, synthetic substitutes.

The early twentieth century was a time of rapid development in the emerging field of endocrinology. Doctors began to understand the way our bodies produce and use hormones to control the various systems and setup of the body. At this time, there was the first division between those who acknowledged hypoadrenia (what we today call adrenal fatigue) and those who did not treat it as a specific condition. Similar to the situation we have today, advocates of adrenal fatigue have argued that the black-and-white boundary between healthy patients and those suffering from Addison's disease was over-simplistic, while skeptics have accused them of merely inventing non-existent diseases.

In 1919, an Italian Professor of Medicine, Nicola Pende, presented a summary of existing research on hypoadrenia. He stated, among other things, that...

> *particularly important are those states of harmonic imbalance which are at the border line between health and disease, and which represent either latent or mild endocrinopathic conditions...It is already understood that for each of the best known hormonal glands, in addition to frank malfunctions there must be recognized minor degrees of perturbation.*

In the 1920's, 1930's, and 1940's thousands of patients were diagnosed and treated for hypoadrenia. However, gradually these diagnoses became less frequent. There was not enough research to identify and diagnose the milder forms of dysfunction of these glands, and their weakness itself was not universally recognized, like the full form of Addison's disease. Endocrinologists focused on diseases and disorders that are were more readily diagnosed and treated. This situation lasted until the late 1990's when the work of Dr. James Wilson, as well as the more accurate cortisol measurement of a patient's saliva, once again allowed doctors to make a diagnosis connected with adrenal fatigue.

Currently, adrenal gland dysfunction, which is not classified as a specific disease such as Addison's disease or Cushing's syndrome, is also described as adrenal weakness, adrenal exhaustion, subclinical hypoadrenia, neurasthenia, or adrenal apathy. However, the most popular description is adrenal fatigue.

The causes of adrenal fatigue

Before you read further, please answer a few of the following questions:

1. Do you often feel tired, shattered, and sore?
2. Do you have a stable level of energy during the day?
3. Do you have a healthy libido and a normal requirement for sex?
4. Do you have an excessive craving for sweet, salty, or caffeine?
5. Do you sleep less than 8-9 hours a day, have problems falling asleep, waking up in the middle of the night, or feeling much more tired than when you went to sleep?
6. Do you feel more awake in the evening, when you should be preparing yourself to go to sleep?

7. Do you often catch upper respiratory tract infections?
8. Do you experience seasonal mood disorders, depression, or memory problems?
9. You have a 'spare tire' at your waistline even though you follow a diet?

If you answered most of these questions affirmatively, this may indicate that your cortisol level is raised and that your adrenal glands are weakened.

As Dr. Christiane Northrup writes – *...the adrenal glands are the main "shock absorber" of the body. (...) They allow you to react to everyday situations in a healthy and flexible way*[1].

The adrenal glands were designed in such a way to quickly react to changes in the internal or external environment of a human being. Usually this is not a problem and they are able to adequately respond to stressors from every possible source – beginning with physically sustained injuries and specific illnesses, to work or relationship problems. However, when the intensity of a stressor increases, and its frequency and duration are prolonged, the adrenal gland becomes weakened; just like a tired horse which stops working altogether without the proper amount of rest breaks, no matter how much we prod him.

Improvised measures such as a cup of coffee in the morning to wake up, a glass of wine, or visiting a gym in the evening to relieve the cumulative tension in the body

---

[1] Dr Christiane Northup – *Women's Bodies, Women's Wisdom. Creating Physical and Emotional Health and Healing.*

will not help. Our biology will begin to reveal more and more somatic symptoms, and permanently elevated levels of stress hormones will be too low as a result. In this way, hyperactive adrenal glands will go into a phase of hypoactivity (they will not be able to produce enough hormones, mainly cortisol)

In spite of the fact that Dr. Wilson's assertion that adrenal fatigue is the result of an already individual stressful situation, it is more often the result of many physical (thermal, chemical, biochemical, metabolic), emotional, or psychological factors acting simultaneously.

A list of the main causes of adrenal fatigue is presented below. It is not an exhaustive and complete list, but it can be estimated that more than 90% suffer from this ailment. Some will find two or three factors in this list that specifically concern them, but in fact, adrenal fatigue can easily be triggered by just one factor.

We should remember (obviously taking into account Dr. Wilson's assertion), that adrenal fatigue is something which appears suddenly. Usually it takes months, or sometimes years, for the glands to find themselves in a state of permanent exhaustion. You also need to remember – which will be discussed later – that adrenal fatigue has four basic phases and various somatic symptoms associated with it.

In one way or another, if we need to identify our symptoms, remember to take a look at the past. Traumatic, emotional, or physical events that occurred over a dozen or several months ago may have been enough for the adrenal glands to gradually begin to lose their strength.

1st Cause – Unresolved stress of an emotional nature

Without a doubt, the first cause of adrenal fatigue is prolonged chronic stress. Importantly, it can come from any area of our lives; regardless of difficulties in a relationship, a rough and surly boss, an unhealthy working atmosphere, moving to a new city, sleepless nights due to colic of a newborn baby, or the long term care of a disabled family member, the result is the same. It is this kind of stress of a relatively small intensity that can be dealt with in the short run, but which can cause serious health effects if it lasts sufficiently long. Stress can also be associated with some unresolved internal conflicts (past or present), a tendency to worry, repressed emotions (anger, guilt, anxiety, fear, or jealousy), depression, or simply a lack of pleasant experiences

2nd Cause – Diet

Diet has a significant impact on the functioning of the hormonal system. There are foods that irritate the body (allergens), hence every appearance of such sustenance on our menu causes a stressful reaction for the body. The most well known allergy-causing agents are gluten, dairy from cows, nuts, chocolate, and seafood.

But they do not only upset our biology. We are currently consuming more sugar than ever before. Two hundred years ago, the average American ate roughly ½kg-1kg of sugar annually, and today it is roughly 75kg! Similar statistics appear in other western countries. Our genes have not changed during this time, so how do our bodies deal with all these empty calories? The answer is clear – we produce additional cortisol (of which one of its tasks is to maintain the right level of sugar) and insulin, which burdens our pancreas and adrenal glands.

3rd Cause – Inadequate sleep

If we go to sleep too late or simply do not care about the quality or length of our sleep, we seriously weaken our ability to cope with daily stress. Our ancestors usually slept about nine hours every night, yet today some of us are able to function sleeping half that time. The average person on average sleeps about six hours, but those who are in the early stages of adrenal fatigue often sleep even less.

Why is sleep so important? A long, peaceful rest at night is exactly what our body requires to be able to re-generate and repair. The body is a remarkable self-healing system, but needs time to make restorative miracles. Thus, we must see to it that we sleep at least 8-9 hours (or longer if you need it), as this will greatly reduce the likelihood that we will suffer from adrenal fatigue. Otherwise, our glands will begin to weaken.

4th Cause – Chemicals and environmental pollution

Each year approximately 2,000 new chemical substances appear on the consumer market in various forms. Some of them go into our food, some into clothing, some into cleaning and medicinal agents, and some into plant protection preparations that we use at home and in the garden. Unfortunately, not all have undergone testing with respect to human safety. All together – the above-mentioned chemicals, environmental toxins (air pollution or chlorine in drinking water) as well as so-called electromagnetic smog (cellular phones, WI-FI networks, transmitters, high voltage networks, etc.) can lead to serious illnesses, compromising various bodily functions. How does this affect our adrenal glands? Well, many of these factors are known for directly affecting the functioning of these glands and the entire hormonal system. Often, our body (especially the remaining parts of the HPA axis) is adaptive for some time to balance this. But, if we constantly and for a longer period of time use harmful substances or are exposed to their unhealthy emissions, adrenal fatigue will be a very likely effect.

5th Cause – Chronic illness

When we discuss prolonged stressors on the adrenal glands, we cannot forget about chronic diseases. Whether we suffer from asthma, arthritis, fibromyalgia, Lyme disease, parasites, diabetes, cancer, or other more or less serious conditions, they are all excessively demanding on our glands. When we suffer for a long period of time, our adrenal glands become overworked and tired not only through stress, which is related to the illness itself or to its physical symptoms (chronic pain), but also to continuous visits to the doctor or hospital, as well as to the use of ineffective drugs and medications.

6th Cause – Trauma

I accurately noted Dr. Alberto Villoldo – *our approach to life is set not in stone but in the nerves of the brain*[2]. It's thanks to these networks that we can tie our shoe, drive a car, and do millions of daily and repetitive activities. Many neural patterns have evolved over the course of human evolution, others are characteristic to us as individuals. Although the main task of neural networks is to assure us of proper functioning and extending life (even during the pre-natal period), connections are created that can cause many problems. For instance, if a pregnant woman is considering ceasing her pregnancy, the neural networks in the fetal brain encode anxiety since the fetus intuitively feels that its own existence is threatened.

This impression of imprinting before birth can put a shadow on the further existence of man. Until man does not consciously change this pattern, a subconscious fear associated with various situations will probably be felt.

[2] Dr David Perlmutter, Dr Alberto Villoldo – *Power Up Your Brain.*

Similarly, when an event – actual or mental – reminds him of a dangerous experience in the past, an instinctive reaction will be triggered and stimulate a specific neural network. Our brain will raise an alarm, and with it will activate the adrenal glands. The more of these internal traumas, patterns, and beliefs we keep in our subconscious and psyche, the more vulnerable we are to the weakening of our glands; which in any case react to the secretion of appropriate hormones. The limbic system can not distinguish a painful event twenty years ago from the recollection of that event triggered by a similar situation in the present, or at least the cascade of thoughts associated with it.

7th Cause – Hippocampus Damage

Lately, scientists are leaning towards the thesis that there is incredible dependence between the brain (specifically the hippocampus) and the adrenal glands. In addition to knowledge on the mechanism of the HPA axis, for quite some time now they have sought a specific place – the "primer" of the adrenal glands, which directly initiates and arouses it. The discovery of this area astonished even the researchers themselves. It was earlier mentioned that the hippocampus – a small structure in the temporal lobe of the brain – possesses many cortisol receptors, thus when the adrenal glands flood the body with this hormone in response to stress, it may become damaged. It turned out, however, that the hippocampus itself is the ultimate adrenal "controller."

The cited Villoldo described it in this fashion – ...*the hippocampus itself regulates the production of cortisol, essentially controlling its own fate.* When the hippocampus is operating optimally, it is able to maintain normal levels of cortisol even in stressful situations. However, if it is damaged – among other things by .... actually excess – it ceases to function as a thermostat, sending information to the adrenal glands about the need to produce cortisol," without a reminder."

The implications of this discovery are enormous as they point to an area that we should pay particular attention to in order to restore equilibrium to weakened adrenal glands.

Other causes of adrenal fatigue worth mentioning:

– excessive physical exercise
– long-term exposure to extreme temperatures
– chronic physical pain
– long-term lack of sunlight
– disturbances associated with the light cycle (shift work, frequently changing the place of residence and continents).

The symptoms of hypoadrenia

When the body is in equilibrium, we are in a good mood. We have a stable level of energy throughout the day, a healthy libido, good resilience, and a positive attitude to challenges that appear. We are pleasantly tired at the end of the day, sleep gives us sufficient regeneration, and our resistance to stress is strong and stable. We do not have cravings for caffeine or extremely salty or extremely sweet foods, and clear thinking and inner clarity make us feel fulfilled, wanted, creative, and productive.

1. A healthy person

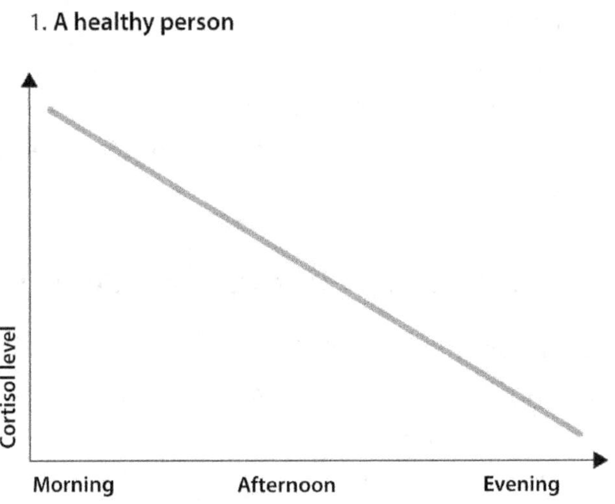

When the level of cortisol is maintained at an elevated level as a result of chronic stress or other causes – as if in a constant mode of readiness for fight or flight – the first symptoms of a disturbance in equilibrium appear. There is a snowball effect, which in biology is referred to as the feed forward mechanism. Elevated levels of cortisol which rise above normal lead to, among other things, sleep disorders, which results in our being more susceptible to stress during the day ... and this in turn again raises the level of cortisol. The consequences of this spiral trigger specific somatic symptoms[3]. They will vary depending on which phase of adrenal weakness we are in. We will discuss this more in the next section.

Here are some of the physical signs of adrenal gland disorder

Difficulty waking up in the morning, even after many hours of sleep

One of the main causes of adrenal fatigue is not enough sleep, therefore more hours of sleep is one of the best ways to recover. However, many people with weakened adrenal glands wake up feeling tired and 'groggy', even though they slept long.

This can be the result of one of two factors. People in the first stages of adrenal fatigue are frequently under a lot of stress, and therefore have distinctly elevated levels of adrenaline and cortisol. This disrupts the natural 24-hour cortisol cycle, leading to alertness in the body, which prevents restful sleep, and a good, lively wake-up in the morning.

People in the later stages of adrenal fatigue will in turn have consistently lower levels of cortisol. However, this translates into much lower blood sugar in the early morning (cortisol , among other things, regulates sugar

---

[3] Bob Wolf – *Paleo Solution, The original human diet* (Published 2010).

in the blood) which results in the body feeling hunger, which forces us to wake up. Many people suffering from adrenal fatigue chronically eat in the late evening or night as a result.

High level of fatigue on a daily basis

In the later phases of adrenal fatigue, the glands are unable to produce sufficient amounts of necessary hormones. This means that the levels of cortisol, along with neurotransmitters such as adrenaline and noradrenaline, are lower than they should be. This relative lack of key hormones explains why patients with weakened adrenal glands find it difficult to do anything or maintain appropriate energy levels during the day. However, there is one exception here (see below) – people with adrenal fatigue often experience an influx of energy in the late evening.

Inability to cope with daily stress

People who suffer from adrenal fatigue have difficulty coping with their daily physical and emotional stress. This is due to the same reasons behind the persistent feeling of fatigue – low levels of stress hormones connected with the later phases of weakening glands.

When we encounter any stress we are dependent on our adrenal glands, which should release adequate amounts of hormones such as cortisol, adrenaline, or noradrenaline. Together with the brain they regulate our reaction to stress and when we need it. They can increase our strength, focus, or alertness. However, when the adrenal glands become exhausted, they have difficulty in secreting the necessary amount of these hormones. Patients with adrenal fatigue often report a lack of enthusiasm, apathy, a lack of interest, irritability, and anxiety.

Craving salty foods

A part of the adrenal glands known as the cortex is responsible for the production of aldosterone, a mineralocorticosteroid that collaborates with the kidneys to regulate the levels of our internal fluids. When the adrenal glands become fatigued, we produce less aldosterone and tend to dispose of large amounts of important minerals in our urine. People with a weakened hormonal system often report frequent urination, which is not uncommon with age, but is actually caused by weakened adrenal glands.

This means that patients with weakened adrenal glands actually lose the ability to balance the level of minerals such as sodium, potassium, or magnesium in their blood. As a result, this leads to cravings for salty food, which supplements the sodium deficiency. If you have an irresistible craving for salty snacks, this may indicate weakened adrenal glands.

Higher level of energy in the evening

Large fluctuations in the daily cortisol profile can cause chaos in our energy level during the day. In a healthy person the cortisol level is highest in the morning – it helps us to wake up, and then, with the passing of the day, it gradually decreases. The lowest is at the end of the day. However, many people suffering from adrenal fatigue (especially in the early stages) experience increased cortisol in the late afternoon and evening. In general, they feel exhausted and weak all day, and suddenly, in the evening, they become revived and energized. Glands are still able to produce significant amounts of cortisol and adrenaline, but this is more a pathological symptom, and is more connected with the active action of the stressor than with normal functioning.

Weakened immune system

Apart from other functions, cortisol possesses an anti-inflammatory effect, which helps guide our immune system. Inflammation is often simply a sign that the body fights the infection naturally, and cortisol takes care that the reaction doesn't spiral out of control. Maintaining a balanced level of cortisol – not too high and not too low – is an important part of this process.

If stress results in elevated cortisol, this anti-inflammatory effect decreases, it effectively limits the proper functioning of the immune system, and can last as long as the cause of the stress lasts. Without a properly functioning immune system, we become susceptible to diseases and infections. On the other hand, excessively low levels of cortisol (further stages of adrenal fatigue) allow the immune system to overreact. This in turn can lead to chronic inflammation and many autoimmune diseases.

Below is a list of symptoms prepared by Dr. Michael Lam[4], a specialist in endocrinology and anti-aging medicine, as well as author of the book *Adrenal Fatigue Syndrome* (2016), which deals with his researching and publicizing adrenal fatigue within the medical community for many years now. In his opinion, hypoadrenal syndrome may be accompanied by any of the following symptoms or ailments. The greater the presence or intensity of these symptoms, the greater the likelihood that adrenal fatigue will affect us:

1. Difficulty falling asleep despite being tired.
2. Waking up in the middle of the night for no apparent reason.
3. Heart palpitations in the night, or when stressed.
4. Constant low blood pressure.
5. Low level of libido and a lacking sex drive.
6. Poor functioning thyroid, often despite taking thyroid medication.
7. Low blood sugar sensation, despite the fact that blood sugar test results are normal.
8. Depression...often there is no improvement after taking antidepressant medication.
9. Endometriosis.
10. Polycystic ovary syndrome.

---

[4] Dr Michael Lam – *Adrenal Fatigue Syndrome* (Adrenal Institute, 2015).

11. Fibroids of the uterus.
12. Breast mastopathy.
13. Hair loss for no apparent reason.
14. Irritability under the influence of stress.
15. Anxiety.
16. Panic attacks.
17. Feeling 'wound up' and an inability to relax. Shivering in the body.
18. Feeling of adrenaline flowing in the body.
19. Inability to gather your thoughts.
20. Inability to cope with even minor, daily stress.
21. Waking up in the morning feeling tired after a restful night.
22. Feeling tired in the afternoon between 3pm and 5pm.
23. Inability to digest simple carbohydrates.
24. Need to drink coffee in the morning and throughout the day to be able to function.
25. Coffee, tea, and energy drinks cause an increase in adrenaline and an adrenal crisis (fatigue, nausea, lack of appetite, weakness, vomiting, abdominal pain, hypoglycemia and hypertension).
26. Feeling tired between 9pm and 10pm, but resistance to sleep appearing before lying down.
27. Hunger for fatty and high-protein foods.
28. Hunger for salty foods such as french fries, chips, and fast food.
29. More than usual dry skin.
30. Hair loss for no apparent reason.

31. Initially physical exercise helps, but then it intensifies fatigue.
32. Hypersensitivity to hair dye chemicals, dishwashing and laundry detergents, nail polishes, and plastics.
33. Hypersensitivity to electromagnetic energy, including cellular phones and computer monitors.
34. Chronic food allergies, especially to dairy and gluten.
35. Inability to conceive, requiring in vitro fertilization.
36. Fatigue and postpartum depression.
37. Recurrent miscarriages during the first trimester of pregnancy.
38. Accumulation of fatty tissue on the abdomen for no apparent reason.
39. Intolerance to temperature, especially hot, and sunlight.
40. Painful menstruation in the absence of periods (amenorrhea).
41. Premature menopause.
42. Constipation for no apparent reason.
43. Joint pain for no apparent reason.
44. Deterioration of muscle tissue.
45. Muscle pain for no apparent reason.
46. Cold palms and feet.
47. Premature aging of the skin.
48. Inability to focus or concentrate.
49. Psoriasis for no apparent reason.
50. Gastritis despite proper gastroscopy results.
51. Lower back pain for no apparent reason; test results are normal.

52. Dizziness for no apparent reason.

53. Weak absorption of fructose.

54. Chronic humming in the ears. Hypersensitivity to noise.

55. Bilateral numbness and tingling in limbs.

56. Recurrent canker sores.

57. Shortness of breath despite having no breathing problems.

58. Ovarian cysts.

59. Breast cancer combined with estrogen dominance.

60. Grave's disease.

61. Chronic thyroiditis, Hashimoto's disease.

62. Feeling of 'heavy legs.'

63. Bruising under the eyes, which does not dissipate after rest.

64. Loss of healthy skin color on the face.

65. Feeling of tension in the whole body and an inability to relax.

66. Postural orthostatic acceleration of heart rhythm.

67. Irritable bowel syndrome more from constipation than diarrhea.

68. Chronic fatigue syndrome which doesn't respond to treatment.

69. Fibromyalgia, which is not resolved after conventional treatment.

70. Systemic candidiasis.

71. Electrolyte imbalance despite proper laboratory results.

72. Irregular menstrual cycle, temporary stoppage of periods.
73. Borreliosis, which does not respond to treatment, or a drug intolerance.
74. Helicobacter Pylori bacterial infection.
75. Problems with memory or concentration.

The list above does not serve as a definitive diagnosis of adrenal fatigue syndrome. It is, however, the first independent step towards determining your state of health, resolving any doubts, or consulting your doctor if necessary. So if there is any suspicion of particular somatic symptoms, reviewing the list may contribute to taking up further action.

IMPORTANT NOTE

Women should care about the proper working of the adrenal glands if they want to gently and painlessly pass through menopause. Weakened adrenal glands are unable to take over the tasks of the ovaries and continue to produce the necessary hormones. If you have "exhausted" the adrenal glands, menopause can turn out to be a bona fide way through the suffering. Women with healthy adrenal glands hardly notice that they are going through menopause ... and that is exactly what it is supposed to be. Hot flashes and other symptoms during this period are not normal simply because they commonly appear.

The four phases of Adrenal Fatigue

As we have seen above, the designation of adrenal fatigues in itself can be misleading as it describes a variety of symptoms that appear on the road to this condition. Fortunately, the majority of people suffering from these weakened glands never goes through the final stages of the disease and often fully recovers from the first or second phase, even though they were not properly diagnosed.

During various stages of the disease, hormone and neurotransmitters levels can fluctuate dramatically. In order to correctly interpret the results of laboratory tests used to detect hormone levels, we need to fully understand the way that certain body's systems interact during each of these phases. Only then can we determine which stage we are in and begin to introduce an appropriate reparative plan.

You can generally say that adrenal fatigue has four phases. They are similar to the stress response phases described by Hans Selye. They are:

1: Beginning of the 'Alarm' phase

Usually it lasts a relatively short time – from a few hours to several days. This stage describes the fast and determined reaction of the body to a stressor(s). It may be an immediate physical threat, or something as simple as a job interview or hospital stay. This can also be a slightly extended situation – a move, a session, a sudden loss of employment, employment probationary period, etc. During this phase, the body is able to produce the large amounts of hormones we need to meet the given challenge. If we were to do testing at this time it would show elevated levels of adrenaline, noradrenaline, cortisol, DHEA and insulin.

During this phase we usually benefit from increased arousal and excitement. We have the resources to deal with the given situation. Nevertheless, our general psychophysical balance and sleep rhythm can suffer from it – temporary fatigue may be noticeable, gastrointestinal disorders, headache, and respiratory infections may occur. People rarely report their symptoms during this phase – in fact many of us enter and leave this first stage many times throughout our lives. If the impact of the stressor passes and no new big challenge arises, the body alone or with little assistance (more relaxation, sleep, supplements, outdoor activities) returns to equilibrium.

2. Continuing the 'Alarm' phase

If it turns out that the stress is not brief and becomes prolonged, the body still needs to reduce its effects. During this second stage, the endocrine system is still well equipped to produce all of the hormones, but the concentration of DHEA and other hormones (primarily sex hormones) may begin to decrease – leading to a DHEA-cortisol imbalance. This occurs because the sources needed for their production are mainly directed to the production of stress hormones.

At this stage, we can start to feel the effects of the excessive effort of the adrenal glands. Usually this will be a larger than normal feeling of fatigue and overwhelming with daily matters, greater impatience, irritability, a propensity for overreaction, or feeling depressed. Our libido falls, problems waking up in the morning appear, dizziness, a feeling of internal shivering. In the evening we may feel completely exhausted. At this point many people begin to develop an unhealthy addiction to coffee, alcohol or other stimulants ... which leads to further instability in the body, as we do not realize the causes of the disorder but only try to eliminate its effects.

2. First, second and third phases of adrenal fatigue

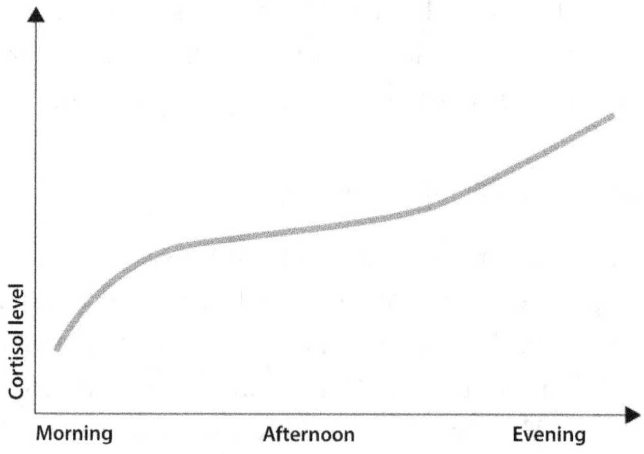

3: The 'Resistance' phase

Stress continues, and the body is still trying to apply adaptive mechanisms. Unfortunately, the adrenal glands begin to have problems with the production of cortisol. Although the ACTH level (pituitary corticotropin, which stimulates the adrenal cortex to produce cortisol) is elevated or high, the body's demands for the amount of stress hormones can not be fully realized. The daily cortisol level is very unstable. In the morning and in the afternoon it is too low, while in the evening it oscillates around the upper limit of normal or it is too high. It aggravates sleep problems – we cannot sleep and sleep is intermittent and does not provide regeneration. The body's immunity decreases and we are more vulnerable to infection and poisoning. The somatic symptoms associated with adrenal fatigue begin to resemble those associated with hypothyroidism – constipation, increased weight, and a reduced tolerance to cold appear. It intensifies a phenomenon known as pregnenolone steal which is the precursor of DHEA, progesterone, testosterone and estrogen. This building block used to produce the above-mentioned hormones is consumed in significant amounts to produce cortisol.

At this stage, a person is still able to function, work, and lead a reasonably normal life; however a hormonal system disorder triggers a significant difference in the quality of life. The resistance phase may well last several months, and several years, more and more intensifying and exacerbating new symptoms of adrenal fatigue.

4: The 'Burnout' phase

After some time (depending on individual predisposition and reserves) the body simply exhausts its possibility of creating stress hormones and the cortisol level begins to be pathologically low. Now, the levels of both sex hormones and stress hormones are low. This condition is sometimes referred to as "burnout" (the term originated with Dr. Fredenberger) and it is what actually occurs when in the end, after a long period of dealing with stress, a breakdown ensues.

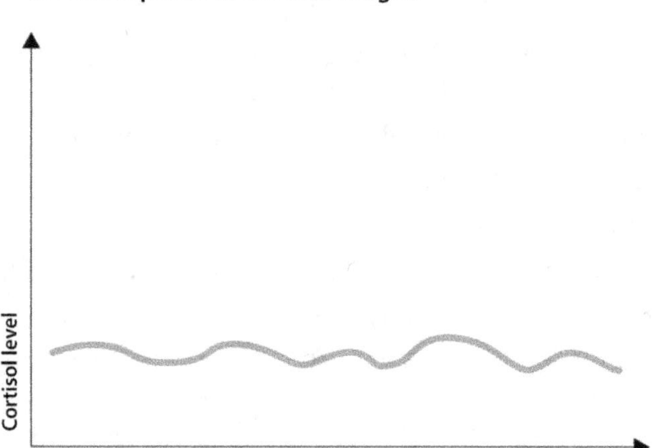

3. **Fourth phase of adrenal fatigue**

All symptoms connected with adrenal fatigue and the degradation of the hormonal system worsen. The parasympathetic system is unable to balance the hyperactivity of the sympathetic system and the adrenal core is continuously stimulated to produce adrenaline. Problems with blood pressure, blood sugar levels, and psychological signs such as anxiety attacks or heart palpitations intensify. An individual suffers as a result of extreme fatigue, electrolyte imbalance, a lack of libido, continual irritation, weak muscles, weight loss, apathy, and a lack of interest in the surrounding world. In fact, this general hormonal inefficiency has serious implications for almost every part of the body. For all practical purposes we have been discussing adrenal fatigue as a disease, whose symptoms aren't much different from full-blown Addison's disease. A way out of this phase of adrenal fatigue requires a long period of time, patience, and often a complete lifestyle change. Thorough consultation and medical assistance is absolutely advised.

CONTEMPORARY MEDICINE AND ADRENAL FATIGUE, DIAGNOSTIC PROBLEMS

Besides cancer, conventional medicine in principle identifies only two dire cases when it comes to adrenal disorders: Addison's disease and Cushing's syndrome – not taking into account their other forms of hypothyroidism. Arguments for and against the existence of adrenal fatigue are now more or less the same as they were eighty years ago. Proponents of diagnosing this affliction claim that dividing the world into people suffering from Addison or Cushing's disease and those who are "healthy" – leaving no room for anything in between – is a flagrant misrepresentation. They also claim that modern laboratory tests use too broad a standard to catch less severe forms of adrenal gland insufficiency and weakening.

Opponents to adrenal fatigue diagnosis, indicate that this is an invented illness, and only because a serious illness (Addison's) exists does not mean that a milder form associated to it must necessarily exist. It is worth noting, the exact same thing was said about hypothyroidism before its milder form of hypothyroidism began to be widely recognized and treated by endocrinologists. Another hypothesis is that medical history is already full of so-called "temporarily fashionable" diagnoses, and adrenal fatigue is nothing more than just that. The counterargument to this is of course the fact that medical books are full of descriptions of diseases that were initially not recognized by the mainstream before they were accepted as actual diseases, requiring diagnosis and treatment.

To show this dual approach, two significant citations are worth mentioning. The first is from the Hormone Foundation, part of the American Society of Endocrinology, which in 2010 wrote:

> *Adrenal fatigue is not a real medical condition. There are no scientific facts to support the theory that long-term mental, emotional, or physical stress drains the adrenal glands and causes many common symptoms.*

The second citation are the words of medical doctor Richard Shames and a riposte to the statement above:

> *Any doctor worth his/her salt understands that the term "adrenal fatigue" means mild adrenal insufficiency. The Hormone Foundation statement readily admits that adrenal insufficiency IS a real diagnosis. To me, they seem to be denying the possibility that some people might have a mild form of a real diagnosis. That's short-sighted and excessively arbitrary.*

Unfortunately, to be treated like a patient, the majority of us must have some sort of serious symptom before we get a doctor's attention. Merely complaining of a lack of energy or decreased sexual drive is usually met with reactions such as "is it transitory depression?" Or "this simply comes with age." On the other hand, when we end up in the hospital with a broken limb or a bacterial infection, we immediately get help.

You must realize that each illness that is recognized by an insurance provider possesses its own code. These codes are defined by the International Classifications of Disease (ICD), which is under the supervision of the World Health Organization (WHO). The latest version of these codes is referred to as ICD-10. The problem is that although Addison's disease (acute adrenal insufficiency) is coded 27.1, yet adrenal fatigue (a milder adrenal insufficiency) has no code. Theoretically, doctors could use code 27.4 – "Adrenocortical insufficiency not otherwise specified," but in practice it is difficult at a time when laboratory tests fall within the "standard range".

Although at first glance it sounds more like a bureaucratic issue, the consequences of the ICD-10 are profound. Without an ICD code, doctors cannot demand payment from the patient's insurance provider. In other words, if they diagnose you with adrenal fatigue, they will not be compensated for treating you. This means that only the more enlightened (as well as less profit-oriented) doctors will consider making such a diagnosis.

Adrenal fatigue is not the only disease that does not fit within the rigid framework adopted by modern medicine. Other examples may be Lyme disease, chronic fatigue syndrome, and candida. Some of them are already actually recognized as real illnesses by Western medicine, but the process for their acceptance was extremely slow. For instance, chronic fatigue syndrome was diagnosed as a disease in 1983, and has been in the Center for Disease Control registry since 2006.

Finally, the last reason why doctors avoid diagnosing adrenal fatigue. In the strict medical sense, it is not easy to treat – a good adrenal fatigue treatment is a change of diet, a lifestyle change, vitamin and herbal supplements, and sometimes hormone replacement therapy. For doctors it is usually easier and more profitable to deal with the specific symptoms instead of the underlying cause. A doctor may prescribe antidepressants or ADHD medications to improve your mood and increase your energy level, while the real underlying physical symptoms will not be taken into account.

To sum it up, it usually takes a long time before the awareness of a newly diagnosed disease penetrates the world of western medicine. Doctors do not devote much of their time to reading the current literature after completing their long and exhausting studies. Often, they are also very curiously interested in diseases that do not endanger the lives of their patients. Fortunately, over time, the approach to adrenal fatigue is changing. As functional medicine and naturopathy become more and more acceptable (for example, currently Canadian naturopaths may write prescriptions, just like medical doctors), adrenal dysfunction is beginning to enter the minds of the medical mainstream. Although it will take some time, it seems inevitable. Thanks to the efforts of such worldly authorities as Dr. James Wilson, Dr. Michael Lam, Dr. Richard Shames, Dr. Christiane Northup, and many others, the knowledge of doctors is constantly growing. For functional medicine and naturopathy, adrenal fatigue is already a commonly recognized ailment that is systematically diagnosed and successfully treated.

Chinese medicine and adrenal fatigue

Traditional Chinese Medicine (TCM) has approached the diagnosis and treatment of a person differently than western medicine. The patient is treated holistically and their problems are not analyzed in the context of dysfunctions of particular organs or systems. The entire biology is an interconnected system of blood vessels, and only that view guarantees greater accuracy in a diagnosis as well as comprehensive health solutions. The terminology and the methodological layer are also different. Dimensions of this study do not allow for detailed explanations; however it is worth noting the approach TCM presents with respect to weakened adrenal glands.

Chinese Medicine (similar to functional western medicine and naturopathy) also indicates long-term stress, diet, macular and micronutrient deficiencies, an insufficient amount of movement, as well as lifestyle and approach to life, as a primary cause of our physical disability. Long-term interfering factors disturb the healthy circulation of energy in the body between the individual organs/systems (elements). According to the so-called Five Phase Theory the adrenal glands are associated with the kidneys (water element). It is their dysregulation (so-called deficiency of right kidney yang energy as well as lack of left kidney yin substances is directly related to adrenal fatigue.) Other main elements and organs associated with them are: the liver-tree, the heart-fire, the spleen – Earth, the lung-metal.

In a very simplified way, here's how it works: In a healthy organism, water hydrates the tree, nourishes it (the essence of the kidneys produces blood accumulated in the liver), and quells the fire to it (the kidneys regulate the functioning of the heart). Wood produces fire by supplying fuel (blood from the liver blood nourishes the heart) and prevents it from overwhelming the earth (the liver stimulates the proper operation of the spleen). Fire creates the earth (the heart gives support to the spleen, providing it with the heat and metabolic energy needed to convert and digest food), transforming matter into the ashes that make up the soil. Fire draws in the metal by firing and melting it (the heart controls lung function). The earth supports the metal (the spleens sustain the lungs, producing the food extract, which connects to the essence of air, creating pure chi (energy) circulating through energy channels), forming minerals and bringing them to the surface, but simultaneously stopping the water by placing a dam in front of it and absorbing it (spleen controls kidney function). Metal invigorates the water (the lungs collect moist chi and pass it on down to the kidneys, which stores the extract by impregnating it with noble substances that reinforce its life-giving properties.) Metal cuts wood (the power of the lung mobilizing balances the power of the liver collecting blood –in this way organizing and suppressing it).

Excessive limitation and control of the circulation of any organ causes its break down and dysfunction; which makes its power and influence weaken, and circulation becomes passive and inefficient. Likewise, exceeding the proper boundaries causes a state of increased activity where the circulation becomes overly intense and rapid.

Imbalance obviously occurs in the case of adrenal fatigue. A weakened spleen (cold-moist type energy) does not have enough power to increase energy in the lungs, and the lungs – in a healthy way, decrease it. Blockages develop in the peristalsis of the intestinal tract, shortness of breath and a propensity for spastic bronchitis, as well as a result of a mucus on the pulmonary alveoli – to various types of asthma. Problems with circulation as well as the operation of the heart ensue (typical symptoms for chronically elevated cortisol). When the earth element (the spleen) is weakened then it does not control the water element (kidney-adrenal gland). The last one directly nourishes the metal, meaning the lung (as well as the large intestine). All together, it causes a weakening of the kidneys.

Disorders of the so-called marrow that is the brain (the vanishing of information transmitted by neurotransmitters as well as disorders in the whole hormonal operation of the body)

In order to restore proper energy circulation, a diet is used which will be selected according to a readout of disorders on the organ-based or function-based meridians and based on heart rate, the appearance of the tongue, as well as objective diagnostics (an interview with the patient). Herbs, as well as acupuncture, will also be recommended with a particular emphasis on lifestyle changes (the ability to relax, contact with nature, and physical exercise such as Qi Gong).

Only a comprehensive approach to the problem gives you a chance of achieving a therapeutic effect on account of the extremely sensitive part of the human body which is the endocrine system as well as the governing of hormones, operation of the brain, and perception of the world.

How to tell if the adrenal glands are fatigued?

The answer to this question is not instantly straightforward and explicit. Of course there are laboratory tests that can be done, but the key is their interpretation. For this you need the assistance of a qualified person who will interpret them correctly. In reality, after laboratory testing (blood, urine, feces, saliva, or whatever) we receive the results along with the standard ranges, but if they are within the normal range, the patient is considered "healthy" and there is no basis to convince the doctor that treatment is needed. The problem is the fact that the standards used are very broad. In the majority of cases, to justify them, simply take a group of the representative population and set the reference range for the two largest deviations from the mean. In practice, this can lead to significant misrepresentations of actual health condition.

Let us take, for instance, the rudimentary TSH (Thyroid Stimulating Hormone) thyroid test. The standard accepted by laboratories ranges from 0.5-5.0 mU/l (in Poland 0.35-4.9 mU/l). As you can see the range is very large – someone with a score of 5.0mU/l has a TSH level 10 times higher than someone with a TSH level of 0.5mU/l and both are recognized as healthy!

Let us look at two hormones whose proper amount is essential for good health, but whose level rapidly drops during adrenal fatigue. These hormones are DHEA and cortisol. During the day the level of cortisol naturally fluctuates, thus the best way to measure it is testing throughout the day. (It is not practiced in Poland itself. Usually, cortisol is tested as well as basic blood and urine tests. – editor's note.) The reference range for cortisol looks like this:

The concentration of cortisol:

- in the morning (laboratory standard):
  0.025 – 0.60 mcg/dL

- at noon (laboratory standard):
  0.01 – 0.33 mcg/dL

- in the afternoon (laboratory standard):
  0.01 – 0.20 mcg/dL

- in the evening (laboratory standard):
  0.01 – 0.09 mcg/dL

You can immediately see the problem The measurement of 0.01 taken at noon will be "normal," and so will the measurement of 0.33, despite being 33 times higher. To put it another way, the cortisol level can drop from 0.33 to 0.01 (a drop of 97%) and it would still be within the reference range. This doesn't make sense and that is why every good doctor or naturopath should define an optimal range rather than simply use the one provided by the laboratory.

The same story occurs in the case of DHEA. The reference range (laboratory standard) for this hormone is usually at the level of 280-640 mcg/dL in the case of men as well as 65-380 mcg/dL in the case of women, but the **optimal level** is much less. In fact the optimal DHEA level is higher than the laboratory standard. Below are examples of laboratory standards as well as optimal levels according to the Life Extension Foundation (LEF)

DHEA for men (reference range):   280 – 640 mcg/dL
DHEA for men (LEF optimal range):   400 – 500 mcg/dL

**DHEA for women (reference range): 65 – 380 mcg/dL
DHEA for women (LEF optimal range): 350 – 430 mcg/
dL**

The above-noted reflections already show that a diagnosis of adrenal fatigue on the basis of one study, standard, or symptom is not possible. To make a proper diagnosis, doctors or naturopaths must rely on multiple tests, sometimes performed several times, and take into account any symptoms which emerge. This requires experience as well as meticulous knowledge of the various systems and relationships in our body, as well as a certain amounts of patience and intuition.

Diagnosing adrenal fatigue should take several forms. First, we have standard hormone testing that involves testing cortisol and various thyroid hormones. These are tests that your doctor will probably instruct you to do. Then, we have research that is more commonly used by naturopaths as well as doctors of alternative medicine – they often examine the levels and interrelations of different hormones and neurotransmitters to have a better notion of how a patient feels. Finally, we have a set of more subjective physical exams which, to a large extent, evolved during the initial period of diagnosing adrenal fatigue.

An accurate diagnosis of hypoadrenia requires a combination of both laboratory tests and patient feedback. Below is a brief description of the principal tests that may be helpful in diagnosing this condition.

Cortisol Testing

To determine your cortisol level, your doctor may order saliva, blood, or urine tests. Currently, cortisol in saliva is recognized as the most accurate result , as it is the most approximate level of this hormone in our cells, meaning this is where the hormonal response actually occurs. A saliva test also has a high diagnostic value since it is a free fraction of metabolites. Remember that it is important to be well hydrated before doing saliva testing – dehydration misrepresents results. As mentioned earlier, individual tests or even a daily average are not enough. The best cortisol test consists of 4 individual tests at different times throughout the day (just after waking up, around noon, then around 6pm, and finally just before bedtime) as well as cortisol level changes in a 24-hour cycle. These levels vary considerably from relatively high when we wake up in the morning and then decrease until they reach the lowest value in the evening. Usually they show approximately an 80% decrease, which is completely normal. Your doctor must see not only the average level of this hormone, but also the morning spike and how quickly it falls during the day.

(In Poland, few laboratories conduct salivary cortisol testing. They can be ordered, for example, on the www.sklep.hashimoto.pl website – editor's note)

Testing involving ACTH

a) Stimulation test

First, basic cortisol levels are tested. Next, the patient is given a dose of ACTH (adrenocorticotropic hormone) in an injection. Then the cortisol level is re-tested. ACTH stimulates the secretion of hormones by the adrenal glands like when we find ourselves in a stressful situation. This test allows an observation of the reaction of our adrenal glands to stress. If the cortisol demonstrates a healthy increase (at least doubled in the blood test) then your adrenal glands are probably in completely good shape. If the spike in cortisol is not very high, it suggests they are weakened.

2) Dexamethasone suppression test

In cases of excessive cortisol synthesis, a doctor may also order a dexamethasone inhibition test to determine whether the excess of cortisol is dependent on the excess production of ACTH by the pituitary gland. The test consists of administering dexamethasone orally (a synthetic glucocorticoid) and assessing the level of cortisol in the patient's blood and urine. Dexamethasone inhibits the production of ACTH, and if the excess of cortisol is dependent on pituitary activity , then the concentration of cortisol should decrease. In this test different doses of dexamethasone are used, usually administered every six hours for two or four days, then samples of the blood or urine are taken for testing.

DHEA Testing

Adrenal fatigue is always accompanied by a reduced production of DHEA, thus some diagnostic conclusions can be drawn on this basis. Testing of this hormone can be done in both blood and saliva. In precisely this case, opinions are divided – some opt for a serum blood test, considering it to be more reliable, while others claim that, as in the case of cortisol, a saliva assessment is of higher cognitive quality.

Blood tests are usually done in the morning – the patient does not need to fast. Usually, two samples are needed for a saliva examination – morning and afternoon.

Thyroid Examination

Surely you are contemplating if a thyroid examination makes any sense when it comes to diagnosing adrenal fatigue? However, this is justified. The complexity of the human body means that one part of the hormonal system (HPA axis) can not exist independently of another part (e.g. thyroid). In reality, there are relationships and correlations between all systems, and weakening in one area easily translates into changes and dysfunctions in another.

In the case of adrenal fatigue, it has been demonstrated that weakening in the hypothalamus and pituitary gland (which belong to the HPA axis) may lead to weakened thyroid function. In other words, if blood tests suggest a slight hypothyroidism, it is very likely that weakened adrenal glands are behind it.

There are many tests that determine the condition of the thyroid, and all of them are blood tests. Similar to the case of examining the level of cortisol, a doctor should not be content with the range of standards provided by laboratories. Actually, it is very common nowadays that someone is diagnosed with hypothyroidism, even if their results are within the standards.

Thyroid Stimulating Hormone (TSH) is produced by the pituitary gland in response to commands from the hypothalamus. As its name implies, the thyroid stimulates the production of T3 and T4, two of the most important thyroid hormones.

The TSH level is inversely proportionate to thyroid activity. If it produces excess T3 and T4, your pituitary releases less TSH (as the thyroid must be stimulated less). Conversely, if you suffer from hypothyroidism, then TSH is likely to be high as your brain is telling your thyroid to produce more hormones. This is the same feedback loop that affects many other hormones, including cortisol.

In people suffering from adrenal fatigue, the thyroid is often weakened, so generally TSH level is maintained at 2.0. Note that the standard range according to laboratories usually ranges from 0.5 to 5.0 mU/l. Here again you can see how important it is to find an optimal level, rather than blindly following laboratory "standards."

Testing blood parameters

To confirm the diagnosis of adrenal insufficiency, it is useful adding some specific parameters during a standard blood test:
– elevated (sometimes also lowered) lymphocyte levels
– elevated or lowered eosinophil granulocytes
– lowered mineral levels – copper, magnesium, sodium and potassium.

Other tests you can do yourself

Testing based on blood pressure

Normal blood pressure is 120/80, which can fluctuate by about 10mmHg depending on whether we are standing or lying down during the test. It may be different when the adrenal glands are weakened. Thus, take two measurements – one when you are lying down and one when you are standing.

Lie on your back and relax for about 5 minutes. Independently, or with someone's assistance, take a measurement. Next, fairly quickly rise to a vertical position and immediately take another measurement. If your pressure is lower after getting up, it can be assumed that your adrenal glands may be weakened. The extent to which blood pressure drops after standing is often proportional to the degree of hypoadrenaline. Of course, this test is just an ancillary method. You need to practice it, because if you are not skilled, the readings may vary dramatically and will not give you a clear picture.

Pupil Examination

You can perform this yourself (using a mirror) or with the assistance of another person. In a dark room, shine a flashlight across the eyes from the side of the face (not directly) of the person and observe the pupils – the pupil should contract as soon as the light reaches the eye. And in that state it should hold the contraction for a long time. In patients with weakened adrenal glands, the pupil will soon dilate (up to 2 minutes). This is related to the balance of sodium and potassium, which is responsible for the reaction of the eye muscles.

White lines on your skin

This test turns out to be true for less than half of those tested, but it is still worth performing. It involves 'drawing' lines on the skin with some dull implement and observing what happens. The line should be white and then red after a while. In people with weakened adrenal glands it will stay white longer before it starts to change.

Body temperature

We take three temperature measurements daily for five consecutive days – roughly three hours after getting up in the morning, then after another three hours, as well as three hours after that. It is important to refrain from measuring after eating or physical exercise. We check the average temperature for all days. It should not fluctuate more than 0.3 degrees (optimally it is about 0.2 degrees). The greater the difference, the greater the possibility of adrenal fatigue.

REMEDIES FOR STRESS, DIET, AS WELL AS A NEW LIFESTYLE – RELIEF FOR WEAKENED ADRENAL GLANDS

Adrenal glands don't have it easy nowadays – everyone can agree on that. However, this elaboration would not be complete if we left the reader with symptoms and difficulties in diagnosing, without providing any tips on strengthening these glands. These include changes in lifestyle, diet, advice on exercise, breathing, and using herbs and supplements. As a rule, forms of self-help do not directly apply to the adrenal glands (although obviously the recommendations will improve their effect) – we are more interested in supporting the operation of the brain, calming the HPA axis, and doing such things that naturally restore normal functioning to the glands and regenerate them. The adrenal glands as such are damaged in the case of cancerous illnesses or diagnosed Addison's disease – defects are then manifested in the structure of the organs themselves. In the other cases, the glands are just certain important processes in the body. Should we improve these processes, the adrenal glands will automatically return to equilibrium.

Undoubtedly, since one of the main causes of adrenal gland dysfunction is a hyperactive nervous system and a brain that is overly stimulated by different types of stressors, we should take a closer look at the different areas of our lives. Either way, stress is a part of it...period. It can not be completely eliminated – besides, there is no need to anyway. We still require certain healthy stimulation to be able to function in today's world, pursue our own goals, and take on various challenges. It is more about stress serving us, rather than weakening us. To make this so, we should know how to neutralize its effects, release it from the body, or simply avoid it. As you will see in a moment, it is also important to change your own attitude towards stress and stressful situations.

We will probably not immediately change our stressful job, but we may start looking for another one knowing that it is generally not good for our health. Perhaps we will not immediately change the tense situation at home or in relationships with other people, but maybe knowing that "taking up the hatchet" does not help anyone, it will drive us to seek new solutions. Perhaps, finally we will not immediately succeed in escaping some serious illness (your own or a loved one) or addiction, yet baby-steps to support the operation of our endocrine glands will initiate an improvement in the functioning of the whole body.

We are aware that the following change proposals are not complete. In spite of that, we hope to inspire readers to further explore the subject independently.

Dealing with Stress

Modern medicine often forgets, or does not take into account, the strength of the mind and the spirit of the body. However, scientific studies conducted over the years show that our psychological state has an actual, measurable effect on our physical health.

Stress is the best example of this. What would seem to be a purely mental state, in fact triggers all kinds of somatic symptoms in our body. These changes affect practically all systems and organs that are so essential for our good health. And, as we now know, serious or long-lasting stress can eventually lead to chronic illnesses like adrenal fatigue.

With this in mind, it seems obvious that the treatment of adrenal gland weakness must include addressing the main causes of stress in our lives. Just as our mental state can bring about illness, an improvement in emotional well-being can and is capable of reversing these ailments. We will describe a few techniques that will assist you in restoring your own emotional and physical health.

It is worth remembering, that in order to heal psychological trauma or any other complicated psycho-emotional disorder, more comprehensive action and support beyond the framework of this elaboration will be required.

First Aid

When a stressful situation suddenly arises, thinking about whether our body will respond or not is meaningless. The body simply reacts, automatically triggering a cascade of related processes. Attempts to stop a reflexive reaction, thinking that getting stressed is not good, will not change what is occurring. As you will read below, your attitude towards such situations is important.

Either way, at the moment of a stressful situation or right after it, we can slightly alleviate its effects. Here's what we can do:

- breathe deeply, inhaling quickly. In exactly this way. Usually, when a difficult emotional situation occurs, we tighten up and stop breathing. It is worth developing a new habit and then when we feel stress, inhale and exhale deeply. Of course, without unnecessary strain.

- take a capsule of good quality B-complex vitamin (preferably of natural origin, not completely synthetic), and one hour before bedtime take 30 drops of valerian in half a glass of water; Drink a cup of melissa or other herbal remedy for calming down;

- go for a 30 minute walk (if the stressful situation is in progress, walk at a faster pace… if it has already passed, walk calmly and breathe deeply);
- jump around like a rag doll several times a day, relaxing the whole body and "shaking" the stress out of yourself; You can also play your favorite music and dance to it ;
- Take a salt bath, immersing yourself up to your neck and lay there breathing deeply, for approximately 15-20 minutes;
- get more sleep, go to bed earlier, take an afternoon nap;
- if the stressful situation lasts several days, organize your time so that in the upcoming weekend you can go somewhere out of town and relax;
- spend more time with nature; forests are especially relaxing, as well as places with flowing rivers or streams
- watch a cheerful, good-humored movie – if you can't choose something, then for 5 minutes simply twist your mouth as if you were really laughing, and then actually laugh out loud for the next 5 minutes;
- Follow the instructions from the "Approach to stress" as well as "Emotions" sections;
- Do not close yourself off to outside help as you may need support from a loved one or professional help.

Approach to stress

The somatic symptoms of stress are very real, and chronic stress should be skillfully neutralized. However, it is important to know that the attitude to stress itself is equally as important. This was shown through an interesting study conducted at the University of Wisconsin-Madison. For eight years the lives of 30,000 American adults were monitored. At the end of each year's study the participants were asked two questions – How much stress they experienced during the period, as well as if they believed that this stress was harmful to them. Next, the data collected, as well as data concerning public death records, were used to examine who from the tested group had passed away, and who was still alive. It was determined that in people experiencing severe stress, the risk of death was as much as 43% higher. However, interestingly, **it applied only to those people who unanimously believed that stress was harmful to them**. In those who truly experienced a lot of stress but unanimously did not find anything harmful in it, their risk of death had not increased. What is more – their risk was the lowest amongst all of the participants in the study (even lower than those who had not experienced severe stress over the past year)

In the end it was estimated that in eight years, about 182,000 Americans (which averages to 20,000 deaths annually) died prematurely – not just from stress alone – but from the belief that stress is harmful. So, can such a change in thinking about stress affect our health and well-being? Science contends, that 'Yes.' By just changing our attitude towards stress, we can change the body's response to stress. How? By remembering and learning that ultimately, stress is not our enemy, but a natural reaction of the body to the challenges we face. This is what researchers did in relation to a study of a group of volunteers. They taught them to think that the body's response to stress is helpful – for example: you breathe faster, through which your brain gets more oxygen, your heart beats faster, so that blood circulates more quickly. Those who actually started to perceive their reactions as positive – *were less tense and more self-confident.* Of course, the reactions in the body did not radically change – but some measurable parameters underwent a change. For example, in a typical response to stress, our arteries contract (studies exist that demonstrate the relationship of stress to coronary heart disease). However, people who themselves developed a different attitude towards stress remained relaxed, despite their pounding heart beat! This information is extremely vital – as it can help us live to a ripe old age instead of a heart attack at the age of 50. As Kelly McGonigal – a stress psychologist – claims, *since we are living in very stressful times, the point is that we "stress better" since the approach to stress is of great importance. If we perceive stress as something positive – which does not mean that we should seek it out or not search for a way out of a chronically harmful situation – the body will begin to believe us and the response to stress will become em-*

pirically healthier[5]. We will develop a so-called biology of courage in ourselves which will allow us to be more resistant to everyday challenges.

INTERESTING FACT

Not everyone knows that one of the stress hormones is also oxytocin – better known as the "cuddle hormone". Pituitary hormones produce it as part of our response to stress, the same as adrenaline, noradrenaline, or cortisol. What is interesting, however, is that in this case the role of oxytocin is to stimulate our motivation to seek support. As claimed by the earlier cited Kelly McGonigal – *When life becomes heavy and full of challenges, oxytocin causes us to begin to surround ourselves with the people we care about. The reaction of the body to stress has a built-in defense mechanism, which is contact with people.* Caring for others, therefore, increases our resistance as well as protects us against the effects of excessive stress and elevated cortisol levels.

Three very effective methods to support the regeneration of the nervous system as well as change our response to stress are presented below:

Silencing the Hypothalamic-Pituitary Adrenal Axis (HPAA)

This exercise is best done when taking a bath or in bed before falling asleep.

---

[5] Keller, Litzeman, Wish *et all 2012 University of Wisconsin School of Medicine and Public Health.*

Lie down comfortably, close your eyes and relax. Throughout the night, take a breath and exhale with your mouth closed. Breathe like this for a few minutes – inhale, count to four slowly, and then exhale while emitting a slight whoosh sound.

After a few minutes, place your right hand just below your navel. Try to also feel a pulse in this area – even though this area is not located near the heart. Realize that precisely this place is connected energetically to the adrenal glands. Imagine that a slower heart rate determines the pace of the operation of your adrenal glands, helping them to slow down and relax. Gently tap the fingers of your right hand on your lower abdomen to keep your awareness on that part of your body. Practice like this for 10 minutes.

As we mentioned above, the DHEA hormone reverses many of the adverse effects of excessive cortisol levels, and assists the body in recovering more quickly after acute stress resulting from some emotional situation, lack of sleep, or excessive physical activity. Research shows that it is possible to strengthen the natural ability of DHEA production by learning to "think with the heart." In other words, it's about choosing thoughts which make us feel better. Here is one such technique proposed by the HeartMath Institute called Cut-Thru (https://www. heartmath.org/).

Concentrating on your heart

Close your eyes, pay attention to your breathing and relax. Observe your current emotional state for a moment. Make yourself clearly aware of what worries you or what is presently causing the tension. Do not change anything, just simply be aware of it and breathe. After a while, direct your attention to the area of the heart (you may put your hand on your chest to help keep your attention there).

Recall something that stirs up a good feeling inside you – maybe a pleasant experience a few days ago, a relaxing walk in the forest, meeting with a close friend, or playing with your pet. This may be something that happened quite recently or many years ago.

Hold this feeling that you have associated with this vision for at least 15-20 seconds. If your mind draws you to the current events, make yourself aware of it and then again, feel good about your vision for a few dozen seconds.

Notice if any internal change occurs. It may be something really subtle. You might also feel nothing. It does not matter. You can return to this practice after some time. Observe when you can perform it more freely – in the morning immediately after waking up, throughout the day during a break, or before bedtime.

It has been empirically found that conscientiously performing this practice can assist in altering the harmful physiological and emotional reactions induced by any kind of stress. Research has shown that after a month of regular practice, DHEA levels increased by 100%, and participants reported increased levels of energy, satisfaction, as well as a significant reduction in anxiety, worry and exhaustion[6].

Inner smile

Thanks to his scientific work, Dr. Lee S. Berk has proven that there is a close relationship between laughter and the body's immune system. Blood tests before and after laughing (comedy films were used in the study) clearly demonstrated a significant increase in the number of natural cells destroying cancer cells and other degenerative cells. Indeed, the body's natural defenses are heightened as a result of laughter. Similarly, in the case of stress. Also, it does not matter whether we are laughing because something actually made us laugh, or we just twist our face in a cheerful grimace for a few minutes, or we simply laugh out loud deliberately. The technique that Taoists have been using for more than 2,500 is presented below. This technique is an "inner smile" and is considered as a way to reduce stress as well as change the body's habitual reactions.

Close your eyes, relax, as well as your breathing, and make sure no one will disturb you for 15 minutes. Grin and hold it for a few minutes. No matter what

[6] Dr Christiane Northup – *Women's Bodies, Women's Wisdom. Creating Physical and Emotional Health and Healing.*

thoughts appear. Keep smiling. Then, draw your attention to the inside of your body, dive right in. Do not strain and do not focus on strength. Just quietly imagine that you are inside yourself. Now, begin a mental journey through the organs and systems of the body. Depending on how much time you have, visit a few or even a dozen places such as the kidney, the liver, the heart, the lungs, the circulatory system, etc. While in each of these places, imagine that the given area has cracked a wide grin. Using your imagination visualize a smiling stomach, brain, or adrenal glands. Have fun with this vision and see how your mood has changed. After a dozen or so minutes of wandering, understand where you are and calmly open your eyes. Let the image of cheerful organs accompany you throughout your day.

Gratitude

You might be wondering what expressing gratitude has to do with adrenal function. Well, quite a lot!

Every activity, action, or method that helps us lower and balance the levels of cortisol (and adrenaline) matters and tips the scale in our favour. Gratitude undoubtedly possesses such ability. It not only allows us to redirect our attention from worries, problems, and challenging situations of everyday life to what we can appreciate, but also strengthens a more positive outlook on life and generates joy. And this has a real impact on the body's biochemistry and well-being.

Below, I will describe the process that I myself regularly use, and I cannot overemphasise how many benefits it brings into my life.

1. Consciously plan to dedicate 30 days to the entire process (of course, you can continue or revisit it at any time).

2. Each day, from the morning onwards, attentively look for things you can be grateful for or appreciate (to remember this, it may be helpful to use sticky notes and place them somewhere visible). Asking yourself auxiliary questions throughout the day can also be helpful – Is there something I can be grateful for right now? Do I notice something I can appreciate? Be thorough and attentive.

Things to be thankful for are usually something mundane and repetitive, as well as what we consider obvious in our daily lives. It doesn't have to be a special occasion or situation (though, of course, it can be). It could be something as simple as a warm bed, fragrant bedsheets, finding a moment for physical exercise, or just stopping to look at the sun. You can also include a child's smile, a brief chat with a neighbour, preparing a delicious meal, or the simple fact that we have eyes and hands, allowing us to see and touch.

I mentioned mindfulness earlier because it is through mindfulness that we will be able to make a special summary at the end of the day.

3. In the evening, before bedtime, write down your observations in a dedicated notebook. It's important that there are at least 20 things you were grateful for during the day. A lot? Believe me, when you get your mind accustomed to searching for new things to appreciate, compiling this list will stop being a challenge. And remembering it at the beginning of the day will make you doubly vigilant not to miss anything!

So, each time (!) starting with the phrase "Thank you for..." (or depending on what resonates with you more: "Thank you to myself for... Thank you, Universe, for... Thank you, life, for... Thank you, God, for..."), briefly write down your gems of gratitude. For example:
— Thank you for being able to do some stretching this morning;
— Thank you for the sun peeking out from behind the clouds for a few moments;
— Thank you for managing to go for a walk despite a headache;
— Thank you for the warm water in the tap.

Of course, as mentioned above, things we are grateful for may repeat.

Every day we can express gratitude for a warm breakfast, a reasonably good sense of well-being, or a functioning car. Important note: we can be grateful not only for things that are obviously good, pleasant or uplifting. We can also appreciate things that are apparently neutral or even harmful or painful for some reason. Yes, that's a higher level of gratitude... but it can open us up to a completely different perception of life. For example, we can appreciate a disagreement with a partner, a headache, a traffic jam on the way to work or a sleepless night. This shows that, in essence, we can be grateful for anything. The choice and perception is entirely up to us.

I can assure you that over the course of these 30 days (and even during them) you will find yourself eagerly looking for little things to describe in the evenings. And this will brighten your life and support your adrenal glands enormously. I myself did not expect, when I first went through this process, that looking back over the year, the 'month of gratitude' would almost make that period of the 12 months 'shine'. I wonder if you will experience similar feelings.

IMPORTANT

Bear in mind patience and gentleness towards ourselves in all of our efforts concerning the reduction of stress and restoration of a healthy physiological response. Remember that the fight or flight reaction is instinctive and has evolved through eons of evolution. Attempts to forcibly reverse the mechanisms associated with it (even if they become chronically dysfunctional) will not bring about positive effects. The amygdala in the brain (midbrain) which is responsible for our reactions of anxiety as well as our response to stress, will sabotage any that are too violent and full of activity. The fear of change (even a positive one) is deeply rooted in the physiology of the brain and, when taken over, blocks every kind of creative potential. In order to "fool" this mechanism, or rather to bypass it, the use of a method of baby-steps is necessary (Japanese technique of kaizen) which on one had will satisfy our need to act, and above all weaken resistance and contribute to the creation of new neural pathways. Only then will this cause our response to stress (outside of truly substantiated cases) to become healthier and free from unhealthy hyperactivity.

Meditation and deep breathing

Scientific studies unequivocally indicate that meditation and deep breathing can change not only the frequency of brain waves, but also circulation and immunological response. They also have a tremendous impact on how we perceive our reality and how we react to it. Meditation takes us from the problem level to the solution level, frees us from negative thoughts, and dissolves old conditioning. It does not deal with any one problem alone, but allows the mind to go beyond the reality of the problems.

For those who are in the 1st or 2nd phase of adrenal fatigue, both meditation and deep, conscious breathing will help to reduce stress, as well as normalize levels of adrenaline and cortisol. This in turn will give the adrenal glands time to rest as well as a much needed regeneration. In people in the 3rd or 4th stages, these techniques will improve circulation, facilitate the elimination of toxins, as well as increase energy levels and increase blood oxygenation.

Here is an example of a meditation exercise connected with breathing:

Make sure nobody will disturb you for the next 15 minutes. Sit with your spine straight and close your eyes. Be conscious of how you feel. Do not change anything just observe. What is happening in the body, in thoughts, in emotions? Do you feel at ease, are you tense? Do you have peaceful thoughts or rather those full of anxiety and irritation? Note all of this. It is actually this awareness that is recognizing all of these things. Also note, that it is not a part of everything you experience ... although it encompasses everything, beholds everything.

After a while, direct your attention to your breathing. Both your breathing and your body are always present — in this actual moment, the moment in which meditation "occurs." Meditation is fully present at this moment, with all that is going on, without involving your attention in thinking, emotions, or bodily sensations.

Observe as your breath flows in and out of the body. Do not control it. Do not change its intensity. Simply observe it as it is at that moment. If a thought interrupts you from observation, just note it and return to your breathing. Practice this for about 5 minutes

Then, to deepen your relaxation even more, repeat several times in your mind – *Everything is in order. Whatever happens, that's how it is... I allow myself feel it.*

Stay relaxed, breathe gently and allow everything, which is the essence of that moment.

After another five minutes, stretch, take notice of the room in which you find yourself, open your eyes and return to your task.

You can practice in this way both morning and evening. It will bring you many benefits even when you are not in a meditative state.

COHERENCE

The content of this section has been adapted from David O'Hare's excellent book: "Coherence Cardiaque 3.6.5." (Polish edition: "Koherencja Rytmu Serca," Cojanato 2023), which I wholeheartedly recommend.

In it, the author describes a valuable breathing exercise which I'll refer to as "3-6-5." The individual numbers signify:

3 – the number of repetitions of the exercise throughout the day;

6 – the number of full breaths (inhales and exhales) per minute;

5 – the duration of breathing in minutes during a single session.

According to the author, heart rate coherence, or harmonising the rhythm of the heartbeat through breath, is one of the simplest and most effective ways to reduce stress, consequently lowering cortisol levels (and balancing adrenal function). This practice is well-documented in scientific research and is recommended by both medical professionals and psychotherapists worldwide.

The effect of a single session lasts in the body for about 4-5 hours, hence the recommendation to repeat the exercise three times a day (first shortly after waking up, second around 12-13, and the last one in the late afternoon).

Procedure for the exercise:

It is incredibly simple. Initially, you may use a timer or dedicated applications (e.g., Breath Ball).

Basically, we breathe in a 5/5 rhythm – inhale for 5 seconds and exhale for 5 seconds. Breathe in through your nose and out through your mouth. This basic rhythm can be modulated slightly, bearing in mind that each inhalation activates our sympathetic nervous system (responsible for mobilisation and action) and each exhalation activates the parasympathetic nervous system, slowing down the heart rate and bringing the body into a state of calm and relaxation.

From the point of view of adrenal regeneration, the 5/5 rhythm mentioned above is the most optimal (it brings balance to the nervous system). However, the 4/6 rhythm (inhale for 4 seconds, exhale for 6 seconds) can also be helpful as it promotes a state of rest and relaxation.

Effects?

They are highly desirable, considering the reduction of stress and everything that overly exploits the adrenal glands. These effects include:

— •   Reduction of cortisol levels

— •   Increase in DHEA levels (a hormone influencing cortisol secretion and slowing down ageing processes)

— •   Increased oxytocin secretion

— •   Strengthening of relaxing alpha brain waves

— •   Enhanced overall sense of calm (as confirmed by questionnaire-based research)

— •   Lowering of blood pressure in cases of mild to moderate hypertension

— •   Decreased levels of anxiety and depression

— •   Improved regulation of blood sugar levels

— •   Reduction of the pathological, chronic inflammatory state in the body

Sleep

It turns out, that sleep restores balance to the adrenal glands better than any other method. It is best to go to bed between 22.00 and 23.00. Sleep before midnight strengthens the adrenal glands much more than going to sleep later, even if you only sleep long enough to ensure an adequate amount of rest. By the way, it is worth adding that it is important that our bedroom be completely dark (no glowing LEDs, clocks, monitors, etc.) Why? Because of so-called porphyrins (complex bioorganic compounds) that create red blood cells, register every kind of light, and transmit this information to the brain. This in turn initiates a disturbance in the activity of a very important hormone responsible for the sleep cycle and wakefulness – melatonin. Incoming light results in us not sleeping as long and as deep as we could. Similar attention should be paid to all sources of electromagnetic energy in the bedroom. Telephones, smartphones, routers, and laptops should be removed from the bedroom and the power supply to these devices should be turned off. If using alarm clocks, let them be traditional devices.

Proper selection of physical exercises

Good physical form serves our spiritual and physical health, but if you suffer from adrenal fatigue, you must be very careful in the choice of exercises. Here are some tips to follow.

1. If you are in the 3rd or 4th stage of adrenal fatigue (thus your energy level is extremely low), you must avoid any strenuous exercises. While jogging or tennis can provide a brief "kick," your hormonal system simply can not allow the production of the hormones which are required by such activity. In other words, after a momentary spike of energy, there will be a rapid "collapse." A better alterna-

tive is walking, Nordic walking, swimming, yoga, Tai Chi or Qi Gong. They will improve circulation and strengthen the body, while not excessively straining the adrenal glands.

2. If you are in the 1st or 2nd phase of adrenal fatigue you can tolerate more demanding and intense exercise such as jogging, weight-lifting, and hiking. In these stages of glandular weakness we tend to have high levels of cortisol, and such vigorous exercise can help to subdue it.

3. Try to exercise in the morning. This will both stimulate your metabolism and later help you sleep well. Exercising in the evening can disturb your natural sleep pattern, which is already a problem for people with adrenal fatigue.

Bear in mind that the length of exercise should depend on your age. Younger people will be able to exercise longer and still retain their briskness and energy. However, with age, our metabolism slows down and it turns out that prolonged exercise really saps our energy. The length of the exercise should be appropriate for your age. One hour of exercise for a young person may correspond to 20 minutes for a person over fifty years of age.

Qi Gong and Tai Chi

This set of health exercises originated in ancient China and links together proper posture, body movement, concentration, as well as conscious breathing. All together, it promotes a healthy flow of vital energy. Both Qi Gong and Tai Chi constitute not only a form of prevention and are helpful in maintaining well-being and vitality, but they are also a means of treatment for many ailments, including those with a psychosomatic background. They are even beneficial for weakened adrenal glands. The healthy effect of Qi Gong was already officially recognized as a therapeutic technique in Chinese hospitals in 1989.

Biofeedback

Biofeedback is an innovative method developed by US researchers in the 1980's with the goal of improving human functioning. It teaches how to effectively manage the working of you own brain and other physiological reactions.

The exercises consist of controlling the course of a game (computer program) with the help of your brain. Information about the operation of the brain is recorded by a small sensor placed on the head of the person doing the exercise. Then the information is sent back to the computer and displayed on a monitor. The person doing the exercise thus has the direct possibility of observing the operation of their own brain, training them, and influencing their work – with just thoughts and attitude, without the use of a keyboard and mouse. They are receiving constant feedback on their progress.

The biofeedback method, in association with relaxation training is becoming more and more appreciated by people living under constant stress and in a rush. Participants report that thanks to biofeedback training they are more peaceful, they sleep better, and they are in a better mood. The effect is long lasting as it is based on the development of appropriate patterns and new neuronal connections in the brain.

Emotions

Speaking of stress and the fight or flight reaction, the subject of emotion cannot be overlooked. In fact, they are either the primer for specific biochemical processes in the body, or they always accompany them. It may be that this surprising situation – such as car accident during a commute – will trigger our emotions (fear, anger, irritation, anxiety, fury, etc.), or just emotions themselves and the thoughts related to them activate our biology, even without the appearance of specific circumstances. You have probably often been apprehensive of some event or meeting, which later never occurred or turned out to be quite tolerable or pleasant. It was enough, however, in order for our imagination to release hormones and let them do their thing as a result of our emotions.

A very interesting concept regarding emotion and connected to stress was presented by Professor David R.

Hawkins[7] – a renowned lecturer and psychiatrist. In his opinion, it is wrong to recognize something or someone externally as a cause of stress. Although, of course, the reaction that the body exhibits is a response to the real or imagined threat of stress that only arises from the pressure of internal tension from repressed and suppressed emotions. It is actually that which causes us to be sensitive to external pressures. From this it follows that the true source of what we call stress is always internal and not external – they are not external factors as we would like to believe, but our personal level of reactivity. As an illustration, Hawkins gives an example that in reality we react with fear, depending on how much fear is already in us. The more fear, the more we perceive the world through a prism of caution and fear. How do you deal with this? Hawkins recommends the Letting Go Technique which he himself devised and thanks to which gives us permission to fully feel our emotions and thereby release the energy behind them. As a result, the blaming of the outside world for our frame of mind disappears and thus we extricate ourselves from the very cause of the stress itself. We are immune to what is happening in our reality and therefore our HPA axis no longer needs to react so rapidly to any potential threat. It is worth learning this process and applying it each day.

---

[7] Dr. David R. Hawkins – *Letting go. The Pathway of Surrender.*

Diet

Proper nutrition is one of the basic defenses against adrenal fatigue. There are two basic things that we must take notice of. First of all, we should avoid all foods that exacerbate the condition of our glands. Secondly, try to eat that which will support a return to health ... and do it in the appropriate way.

1. Identifying allergies, hypersensitivity, and food intolerance

Why is food hypersensitivity such an important issue if you have weakened adrenal glands? The point is that they prevent our bodies from absorbing and using their nutrients, which we need, and encourage inflammation and disturb our sleep/wake cycle as well.

Food allergies, hypersensitivity, and intolerance impede proper digestion and excretion in our intestines. That is why diarrhea, constipation, as well as other intestinal problems are often the first sign of food intolerance. They stop the optimal absorption of food, causing a weakening of the body and low energy levels. They contribute to the formation of intestinal inflammation which triggers the secretion of histamine (along with their typical symptoms of sneezing and coughing). Moreover, if we do not digest properly, harmful bacteria proliferate in our intestines which further weakens our immune system.

Here are some simple ways to deal with food intolerance and sensitivity.

- Do blood tests to find out if you are allergic, get tested with devices that use bioresonance (e.g. vega-test) or order home tests (e.g. Food Detective). Unfortunately, no test is 100% reliable, so only treat the results as indicators, based primarily on your body's own response. If you are not sure, you can try to eliminate one thing for a period of time, for at least a week, until you identify the "culprit." Either way, avoid uncertain or questionable food.

- Use substances that strengthen the intestines. The most well-known supplement in this category is glutamine – an amino acid whose cell walls your intestines use as a source of energy. It helps in the repair and regeneration of the intestinal epithelium. Sodium butyrate also works perfectly, as it is the basic "food" for colonocytes – intestinal epithelial cells that are responsible for the reconstruction of this section of the digestive system. This substance helps: reduce the permeability of the intestinal walls and maintain its integrity, stimulate the production of mucus, which is a mechanical protective barrier for the intestinal epithelium, prevent the entry of dangerous microorganisms into the digestive system, reduce stomach ulcers, increase the number of villi cells in the ileum, accelerate the regeneration of the intestinal mucosa fat.

You can also try herbs that alleviate irritation such as licorice root or red elm that cover the intestinal epithelium and protect it from inflammation.
— Take supplements that improve digestion. If you have digestive problems and you experience symptoms such as bloating, gas, diarrhea, or constipation, it may be helpful to ingest probiotics or digestive enzymes. They facilitate digestion and better absorption of nutrients from food.

2. Follow simple rules for eating

Because everything in our bodies works on the principle of interconnected vessels, anything that increases stress in the body – undoubtedly including what we put into our mouths – contributes to increased cortisol production, which, of course, weakens the adrenal glands. There is an interesting correlation here regarding the levels of cortisol and blood sugar.

Overproduction of cortisol due to excessive external stress leads to an increase in blood sugar levels. Chronic stress can lead to insulin resistance, type II diabetes, metabolic syndrome and increased inflammation in the body.

Similarly, negative effects occur in the "reverse direction." Various internal factors, including a diet rich in processed products and a high carbohydrate content, influence increased cortisol production. These factors cause excessive spikes in blood sugar.

So, what constitutes an anti-stress diet that supports the adrenal glands? Here are some useful and practical tips.

— Maintaining a normal blood sugar level is essential to prevent energy crashes and excessive cortisol production. Therefore, in adrenal exhaustion and chronic stress, opt for foods with a low glycemic index or ensure that your daily glucose curve is essentially flattened (to avoid unnecessary sugar spikes). Here, I encourage you to turn to an excellent resource on this topic, which I consider one of the most important health books in recent times. It's "Glucose Revolution" by Jessie Inchauspe.

Its inestimable value lies in the fact that it does not promote any particular diet as superior to others. Instead, it focuses our attention on maintaining stable blood glucose levels through a few simple recommendations.

Some of these include:

— taking food in the right order. And this is not about the previously known recommendations of dividing meals due to the ease or difficulty of digesting individual ingredients (e.g. proteins together with carbohydrates are digested worse, and proteins combined with vegetables – better). This approach is more about ensuring that each meal (mainly the one that contains a lot of carbohydrates) start with a green snack or vegetables containing fiber, because this is what can keep post-meal blood sugar spikes in check. It turns out that if carbohydrates from cereals or high-starch products land in the stomach first, they will quickly reach the intestines, where they will be broken down into glucose molecules, and getting into the blood will cause a significant spike in sugar. Interestingly, however, if we first eat vegetables with a high amount of fiber, e.g. cooked broccoli or Brussels sprouts (or a vegetable salad), the situation will be completely different and the glucose curve will remain flat. The length of breaks between individual meal components does not matter. So, right after vegetables or salad, we can move on to proteins or carbohydrates.

— Consuming so-called savoury (protein and fat-rich) breakfasts without the addition of carbohydrates or with a small amount of them. The idea is not to further boost cortisol levels. In the morning, cortisol levels are usually higher because the body is preparing for activity after a night's rest. As we know, cortisol levels rise if blood sugar levels increase, and this will happen after a carbohydrate-rich meal (e.g., porridge, oats, cereal, sandwiches). Hence the recommendation to keep breakfast protein and fat-focused (e.g., bacon and goat cheese omelette, vegetable omelette, mozzarella in a pan with olives and tomatoes, soft-boiled eggs with pickles and avocado, etc.) Moreover, as Jessie Inchauspe write:

A breakfast that causes a big spike will make us hungry again soon. What's more, such a meal will disrupt our blood sugar levels for the rest of the day, so lunch and dinner will also cause significant spi-

- Avoiding eating "naked" carbohydrates throughout the day. As often as possible, precede them with some green snack, apple cider vinegar, or something with fibre that will prevent rapid glucose releases into the blood.
- Movement after meals. If we sit in a chair or return to our desk immediately after a meal, glucose will accumulate and cause a noticeable spike in blood sugar. However, if we perform a few simple physical exercises, our muscles will almost instantly utilise glucose, preventing its accumulation and avoiding a sugar spike. What exercises can you do? A 20-minute walk outdoors is excellent, but if space is limited, do at least 30 squats or 30 calf raises in a standing position

Fasting

Not only does a healthy diet have a significant impact on our adrenal glands, but regular abstention from eating also plays a crucial role. Particularly recommended forms of fasting (which are becoming increasingly popular) are the so-called intermittent fasting, characterised by appropriately timed eating windows. The most effec-

---

[8] Jessie Inchauspe – Glucose Revolution. The life – changing power of balancing yout blood sugar.

tive ones are 14/10 or 16/8. These denote fourteen or sixteen hours that elapse from dinner to breakfast, along with the period in which we should consume meals – ten and eight hours, respectively. As research indicates, these designated fasting periods strongly support the body's regeneration and the recovery of individual organs (including the adrenal glands). This has a doubly positive effect as it aligns with the overnight rest period.

In the case of adrenal exhaustion, regular 24-hour fasts are also recommended, as they further promote the activation of the body's repair mechanisms. Longer fasts, although beneficial to health, are not particularly recommended in stages III or IV of adrenal insufficiency.

For more useful information on fasting, you can refer to Dr. David Jockers' book: "The Fasting Transformation"

Limit caffeine

Caffeinated drinks can improve your mood for a short time but, by the way, remember that they put a lot of stress on our adrenal glands and the hormonal system. Caffeine stimulates the adrenal glands to produce adrenaline and cortisol in exactly the same way as when they are under the influence of the fight or flight reaction. Over time, since the glands become weakened, they have less and less ability to react in this way. People struggling with adrenal fatigue often say that "coffee doesn't work for me" – most often because of the fact that continuous stimulation has weakened their glands so much that they are no longer reacting properly.

Giving up that morning cup of coffee, tea, or caffeinated beverage can be and sound scary, but is an important part of your recovery. Many of us experience short-term symptoms of caffeine withdrawal, though they generally go away within a week. After giving up caffeine, most people with weakened adrenal glands report having higher, sustained levels of energy during the day, without any rapid spikes or drops caused by caffeine.

If you absolutely cannot give up coffee, use a roasted grain beverage or boil ordinary coffee (a few minutes boiling coffee over low heat with the addition of a pinch of cinnamon, cloves, or cardamom will completely change its makeup – it then becomes a strengthened, deacidified drink used for decreased immunity, migraine pain, and stomach weakness)

Keeping properly hydrated

This is a simple but basic recommendation. Good hydration is important for everyone, but if you suffer from adrenal fatigue, it is doubly important. When speaking of hydration we mean drinking pure water during the day, without any other fluids. We can go one step further by adding a pinch of sea salt or Himalayan salt to our glasses, or a few drops of lemon. Many people with adrenal fatigue have a deficiency of minerals and electrolytes. Water should be at least room temperature, but warm water or very warm water drunk in small sips is significantly better.

Superfoods for individuals with adrenal fatigue

In addition to foods you should avoid, another certain group of products exists which can actually help you recover from adrenal fatigue more quickly. They include — cruciferous vegetables: broccoli, cauliflower, brussel sprouts, cabbage, kale, as well as celery, spinach, onion, asparagus, avocado, arugula, beet, lettuce, parsley, seaweed, coriander, basil, thyme, olive oil, blueberries, goji berries, and fermented foods.

VITAMINS, SUPPLEMENTS AND HERBS – ADDITIONAL REGENERATION FOR THE ADRENAL GLANDS

Additional supplementation with the goal of strengthening weakened adrenal glands will serve, above all, to restore proper functioning to the body as a whole with reference to the brain (hippocampus) as well as the nervous system. As a result, overloaded adrenal glands will also be able to return to equilibrium.

The recommended measures have been divided into three groups. Listen to your own body. Your instinct will tell you how to compose your own set of supplements, while taking the following tips into account. At the same time – chronically ill people, pregnant women, as well as breastfeeding mothers should consult a doctor or pharmacist when determining the correct dosage.

Most important

- **Vitamin B-complex** – 100 mg 1× daily + extra Vitamin B5 – 100 mg 1× daily (the adrenal glands do not function properly without these vitamins)
- **Vitamin C + bioflavonoids** – 1000-4000mg daily in separate doses
- **Omega 3 oil** – 1000-5000mg daily (nourishes the brain and regenerates the hippocampus, calms the fight or flight reaction) Nourishes the brain with omega-3 fatty acids, will quickly regenerate the hippocampus. As claimed by Dr. Alberto Villoldo – *After only six weeks of an increased supply, you will begin to notice beauty where until now you have only seen ugliness and sense the possibilities in that which you solely perceived as a threat*[9]. The hippocampus regenerates quickly and when we cease nourishing our brain with adrenaline, cortisol and ... caffeine, we will begin to liberate ourselves from the negative effects of stress.

Extraordinary stories about the positive impact of omega-3 oil on the regeneration of the nervous system and the reduction of stress, thus balancing cortisol secretion, can be found in Dr. David Servan-Schreiber's book – "The Instinct to Heal: Curing Depression, Anxiety, and Stress Without Drugs and Without Talk Therapy".

---

[9] Dr Alberto Villoldo – *One Spirit Medicine* (Astropsychology Studio, 2015).

Among other things, the author describes the cases of two men suffering from long-term psychological and emotional problems. The first, a 35-year-old manager, struggled for many years with bipolar disorder, which was resistant to all forms of traditional therapy. A turning point in his illness was an experimental method of taking 9 cod liver oil capsules a day (3 times 3 capsules before meals). Within a few weeks, his psychological symptoms had almost completely disappeared and he was able to enjoy the inner balance he was looking for.

A similar story involved a young teenager who had been plagued by overwhelming anxiety, depression and suicidal thoughts for several years. In this case, conventional therapy with antidepressants had no effect. Electroconvulsive therapy was even considered. Only by taking several grams of cod liver oil a day did the suicidal thoughts disappear completely within a few dozen days. The young man stopped feeling uncomfortable in public places and started sleeping well again. After nine months, all the symptoms of years of depression were totally gone.

Important

Theanine – it calms, reduces stress and anxiety, and stabilizes mood. It assists in achieving a state of tranquility – deep relaxation while simultaneously maintaining vigilance of the mind. It stabilizes an optimal blood pressure. Assists in dealing with insomnia. We start with a small dose on an empty stomach and increase it to one which will allow you to loosen up (usually in the range of 200-400mg daily).

GABA (both an amino acid and neurotransmitter with a calming and relaxing effect). It can be successfully used in problems associated with situations of anxiety, thought disorder, and physical tension. Causes a state of decompression and relaxation, stimulates the regeneration of gastrointestinal tract epithelial tissue, and intensifies regenerative and restorative processes. With low blood pressure we must take care in its use. We take doses of 500mg-1500mg on an empty stomach about 30-60 minutes before going to bed.

Taurine (a helpful amino acid in issues related to anxiety and emotional destabilization. It really helps in limiting reactions of agitation and restlessness, while at the same time does not cause numbness. Usually a dose of 1000-2000mg daily on an empty stomach is sufficient (similar to the case of GABA, exercise caution regarding dosage, if you have a considerably lowered blood pressure).

Coenzyme Q10 (or better yet, its better bioavailable form – ubiquinol) – 50-100mg 2x daily.

Glutathione – regarded as one of the most effective antioxidants – it neutralizes the action of free radicals responsible for inflammation in the body and brain – daily dose of 250 mg – 1-2x

Magnesium – 300-800mg daily in half doses (best in chelate form of fumaric acid, citric acid, glycinate, or malic acid) – it increases the elimination of magnesium in urine at times of elevated cortisol, thus it is important to remember this supplement.

Alpha-Lipoic acid – helps in removing toxins from the brain, a powerful antioxidant – 300mg daily.

Turmeric (in the form of curcumin) – raises superoxide dismutase (SOD) levels as well as glutathione: two antioxidants important for the brain's functioning and regeneration.

Zinc – 15mg daily (in ionized form or amino acid chelate).

Selenium– 200-400mcg daily

Cod-liver oil – 1-2 teaspoons in the case of children, and 1-2 tablespoons for adults.

Adrenal concentrate.

A good way to support the recovery of exhausted adrenal glands is to use liquid or powdered bovine adrenal concentrates. Of course, only raw materials from free-range animals with access to fresh grass are used for this purpose. No growth hormones, antibiotics or pesticides are used during breeding. How to use a given preparation can be found on the leaflet

Complementary (but no less important)

In addition to mineral supplementation, the use of adaptogens will be essential to restore proper adrenal function. Their extremely useful effect is that, thanks to their properties, they allow the body to return to psycho-physical balance, regain strength after exhausting situations, and balance the level of cortisol secreted, which is of great importance in the case of weakened adrenal glands. This means that adaptogens should be included in all activities and treatments aimed at restoring the proper functions of these organs. Of course, there is no need to use all adaptogens at once, especially since the amount of them currently available on the market is quite large. Just include 1 or 2 types in your daily diet and use them for 3 months or observe your well-being during the treatment and replace them with others to find those that work best for you. Below are several types of popular adaptogens that have a beneficial effect on the regeneration of weakened adrenal glands.

Maca – It adds energy, increases endurance and resistance to stress, recommended for states of physical and mental exhaustion The recommended dose is 1,000 to 3,000 mg (1-3 g) of maca root daily.

Safflower beetle (leuzea) – It is used as an aid in chronic fatigue, weakness, reduced immunity and functional disorders of the nervous system Recommended dose – in powder form: 1-2 teaspoons 2x a day, alcohol extract: 3x a day 1ml

Cordyceps – It fights stress and fatigue and naturally increases energy levels. Increases physical performance and libido. Dosage – usually 500mg to 4g per day

Chinese Schisandra – like other adaptogens, it helps maintain cortisol at an optimal level, protects nerve cells and increases the amount of neurotransmitters (including GABA), i.e. substances that transmit signals between cells of the nervous system Dosage: usually 200 to 1000 mg of schisandra is used daily.

Astragalus (trabeculae) – strengthens the immune system, is recommended for people who are fatigued and ill, strengthens adrenal gland operation – about 500mg daily.

Siberian ginseng – recommended for hormonal disorders, increases the adaptive ability of the body as well as tolerance to stress, increases psychophysical performance (not recommended for people suffering from hypertension, pregnant women, as well as people suffering from heart disease) – 500mg 1x daily before 5 pm.

Ashvaganda – strengthens the nervous system – has a calming and quietening effect, regulates the hormonal system – improves thyroid function as well as the adrenal glands, stimulates the immune system as well as the blood – (250mg 2-3 times daily).

Mountain Rose – Adaptogenic herb, recommended for people with physical or mental exhaustion, increases resistance to stress, acts as an antidepressant, prevents brain degeneration (200mg 2-3x daily)

IMPORTANT NOTE – USE OF DHEA

Of course, as far as possible, it is best to naturally restore the proper functioning of the adrenal glands. If you don't get the desire result, you may want to consider DHEA biohormone supplementation until your health improves. High doses of DHEA taken for a longer period is not recommended as it can significantly affect daily cortisol fluctuations, but lower physiological levels are recommended most for restoring normal hormonal levels. Begin with the lowest possible dose – most people take 5-10 mg twice daily, others take 25mg in two doses. DHEA is generally well tolerated but in the case of women there may be side effects in the form of acne. This can be prevented by taking a DHEA metabolite called 7-keto-DHEA (practical doses are about 50-100mg daily). After about 3 months, it is good to check if DHEA levels have returned to normal and then limit supplementation. If you think you would like to supplement DHEA, you should do so in cooperation with a doctor or certified naturopathy who is experienced in this type of therapy.

OTHER TOPICS

Mitochondria functioning and the condition of the adrenal glands

Mitochondrial medicine is still in its infancy in public awareness, and yet everything depends on the functioning of mitochondria (tiny cell organelles) responsible for the process of creating energy in the body. Also adrenal function.

As with other body systems and mechanisms, the principle of reciprocity applies here

On the one hand, cortisol produced by the adrenal glands – especially if its amount is chronically elevated – will have a destructive effect on the condition of mitochondria, of which quite a lot are contained in adrenal cells. On the other hand, the weakening of mitochondrial functions will adversely affect the adrenal glands and it will be difficult for them to return to balance.

Here are some thoughts on the relationship between the adrenal glands and mitochondria

1. Cortisol levels have a significant impact on mitochondrial function through various mechanisms.

Glucose metabolism: Cortisol can affect glucose metabolism by increasing glucose levels in the blood. High glucose levels can lead to changes in the energy metabolism of cells, including mitochondria, which are the main place of energy production in the form of ATP. Long-term increases in cortisol levels may lead to mitochondria overload and disruption of their functioning.

Oxidative stress: Excessive secretion of cortisol can lead to increased levels of oxidative stress in cells, which can damage mitochondria. Excessive deoxidation may lead to damage to mitochondrial membranes, mitochondrial enzymes and mitochondrial DNA, which in turn may impair mitochondrial function.

Mitochondrial gene regulation: Cortisol can influence the expression of genes related to mitochondrial function by regulating the activity of appropriate signaling pathways in cells. Disturbances in the regulation of mitochondrial genes may lead to disorders in the functioning of mitochondria.

– **Aging of the body:** High cortisol levels can accelerate the aging process of cells, including mitochondria. Mitochondria are particularly susceptible to damage related to oxidative stress, which may lead to a deterioration of their function with age.

2. How does mitochondrial health affect adrenal function and why is it important to take care of your mitochondria?

Energy production: Mitochondria are the main site of energy production in the form of ATP. High energy efficiency is necessary for the proper functioning of the adrenal glands, which are responsible for the secretion of many hormones, including cortisol, aldosterone and adrenaline. In cases of mitochondrial failure, an energy deficit may occur, which may negatively impact the ability of the adrenal glands to secrete hormones.

Stress resistance: Mitochondria play an important role in regulating the body's response to stress. Stress can lead to increased energy demands, and healthy mitochondria can provide the energy needed so that the body can deal with stress effectively. Mitochondrial disorders can impair the body's ability to adapt to stress, which may negatively impact the functioning of the adrenal glands and their ability to secrete hormones.

Reduction of oxidative stress: Mitochondria are the main site of production of reactive oxygen species (ROS), which can damage cells, including adrenal cells. Mitochondrial disorders can lead to overproduction of ROS and increased oxidative stress, which can lead to mitochondrial damage and deterioration of adrenal function.

Regulation of metabolism: Mitochondria play an important role in metabolism, including the metabolism of glucose, fats and amino acids. Mitochondrial disorders can lead to metabolic disorders that can negatively impact the health of the adrenal glands and the entire body.

Since mitochondrial function is the subject of my second book (scheduled for release in 2024), I will not expand on this topic further. You will find helpful tips in the various resources available on supporting mitochondrial function as one of the strategies to restore balance to the exhausted adrenal glands.

How long does it take to recover from adrenal fatigue?

This is one of the most frequently asked questions by people suffering from hypoadrenia. Unfortunately, the answer is not so simple and clear-cut. Generally, it will take about 6 to 18 months, but it depends on the individual. For some it will last less than 6 months, for others it may stretch for up to two years before the adrenal glands truly return to form.

Individual return to health is related to several factors. First, it depends on the severity of the condition in which the person finds themselves. If this is the first or second phase, the return to equilibrium should be relatively short. If the disorder was caused by temporary stress at work, a fleeting illness of a loved one, or bereavement, it can be assumed that elevated cortisol levels will return to normal after the stress has subsided. In fact, many of us experience the first or second stage of adrenal fatigue several times throughout our lives and emerge from it in a few weeks or months when its cause disappears.

When a person is in the third or fourth stage of hypoadrenia, treatment will of course take longer. In these stages, both the adrenal glands and the entire hormonal system are severely agitated and weakened, and the production of at least several hormones is extremely unregulated. To rebuild strong adrenal glands, it is vital to introduce radical lifestyle changes, a proper diet, as well as proper supplementation. It takes time and presumably such a process will last for at least six months.

For people, who for some time find themselves in an extremely grueling fourth phase where both sex and stress hormone levels have decreased significantly (indicating a considerable weakening of the glands), treatment will take even longer. You should expect therapy lasting at least 12 months, which may also, in addition to changes in lifestyle, diet, and supplementation, require the need to take hormones ordered by a doctor.

As is the case with most diseases, much depends on the patient themselves. No matter how good the recommendations are from your doctor, if you do not follow them, it's difficult to expect optimal results. For instance, if someone with adrenal fatigue continues to eat junk food, will not exercise (or overloads exercise), will not take the proper supplements, then their treatment will certainly take much longer. On the contrary, a person who follows the advice of a doctor or a naturopath can expect quicker and better results.

This not only applies to lifestyle and dietary choices. As far as possible, patients should recognize and eliminate the source of their stress. It is sometimes difficult, but it is an essential part of a healthy recovery. Toxic relationships, overly stressful work, family quarrels, or financial troubles – should somehow be eliminated or even toned down. Often, after resolving these problems, patients experience great relief, as if they have taken a heavy weight off their back. It also means that their adrenal glands and the entire HPA axis have gotten rid of a great dose of stress.

Taking care of each stressor in turn is the best approach. Recognizing what makes us happy and stressful is easy, then the hardest part begins – making the necessary changes. They are often associated with a fundamental change of views and perspectives. For example, if a well paying job is ruining your health, will you get off the corporate ladder and return to a simpler, more satisfying life? If a relationship has been the cause of your stress for many years, do you dare end it and start life over? All of these kinds of problems can be successfully resolved with the support of family, friends and perhaps, a good therapist.

SUMMARY

An epidemic adrenal fatigue is spreading throughout the developed world. What is its most obvious indication? A chain of coffee shops popping up at a quickened pace! In fact, on every street corner you can identify a direct link between stress and adrenal fatigue, and Starbucks or Costa Coffee. Stimulants like coffee are the simplest way to mask our exhaustion, but in reality, they just conceal the problem.

You can become addicted to excessive stimulation – or more precisely, from the chemicals produced by their release. It is also easy to mistake vitality with the daily pursuit for adrenaline. The difference is that vitality is rejuvenating, whereas the flooding of the body with stress-related chemical compounds leads to burnout, tissue damage and, among other things, adrenal fatigue.

Modern civilization forces us to live under constant pressure – time, deadlines, contracts, and commitments.

It causes a constant rush and a lack of relaxation. The daily to-do list never gets shorter. We have to pay in installments, follow the norms ...always doing something. This applies to everyone – young and old, rich and poor, men and women, pensioners, active professionals, and students.

However, we must find the time to rest. Who knows if this is not the top priority of our cortisol times. From the beginning of evolution stress has forced us to develop creative solutions or adaptations. It is no different nowadays – in the face of modern threats to civilization our species must face the next challenge for survival. Otherwise our bodies simply refuse to obey us... we will grow older, get sicker and die faster and faster, instead of enjoying good health into our old age. It is worth changing your lifestyle and creating within yourself a new approach to stress. It is worth paying more attention to everything that we put into our mouths. It is worth finally taking care of rest, silence, and relaxation each day. Our bodies and our adrenal glands will be grateful to us.

BIBLIOGRAPHY

Lothar Ursinus – *Mein Blut sagt mir...*

Dr Rick Hanson, Dr Richard Mendius – *Buddha's Brain*

Nora Gedgaudas – *Primal Body Primal Life, Beyond the paleo diet for total health and longer life*

Walter Hartenbach – *Die Cholesterin-Luge, das Marchen vom bosen Cholesterin* (The cholesterol lie, the myth of bad cholesterol, ABA Publishing House, 2010)

Jon Kabat Zinn – *Full Catastrophe Living. Using the Wisdom of your Body and Mind to for Stress, Pain and Illness*

Jean Carper – *Your Miracle Brain*

Dr Christiane Northup – *Women's Bodies, Women's Wisdom. Creating Physical and Emotional Health and Healing*

Dr David Perlmutter, Dr Alberto Villoldo – *Power Up Your Brain*

Dr Alberto Villoldo – *One Spirit Medicine*

Charlotte Watts – *The De-stress Effect: rebalance your body's systems for vibrant health and happiness*

Jessie Inchauspe – Glucose Revolution. The life – changing power of balancing yout blood sugar.

Dr David Servan-Schreiber – The Instinct to Heal: curing depression, anxiety and stress without drugs and without talk teraphy

David O'Hare – Coherence cardiaque 3.6.5

Dr David Jockers – The Fasting Transformation. Burn Fat, Heal Your Body & Transform Your Life

Dr Daniel G. Amen – *Change your brain, change your body, use your brain to get and keep the body you have always wanted*

Bob Wolf – *Paleo Solution, the Original Human Diet*

Dr Michael Lam – https://www.drlam.com/articles/adrenal_fatigue.asp?page

Dr Michael Lam – *Adrenal Fatigue Syndrome. Reclaim your Energy and Vitality with Clinically Proven Natural Programs*

Monika Skuza – *Adrenal fatigue w funkcjonalnym modelu* (Adrenal Fatigue Functional Model) http://www.tlustezycie.pl/2014/10/wyczerpanie-nadnerczy-w-funkcjonalnym.html

Monika Skuza – *Samodzielna diagnostyka wypalenia nadnerczy* (Self-diagnosing adrenal fatigue) http://www.tlustezycie.pl/2013/03/samodzielna-diagnostyka-wypalenia.html

Monika Skuza – *Gdy stres nie pozwala ci wyzdrowieć (When Stress doesn not allow you to recover)* http://www.tlustezycie.pl/2014/06/gdy-stres-nie-pozwala-ci-wzydrowiec-lub.html

Kelly McGonigal, Ph.D – *How to Make Stress your Friend* http://www.ted.com/talks/kelly_mcgonigal_how_to_make_stress_your_friend?language=pl

Dr David R. Hawkins – *Letting go. The Pathway of Surrender*

Robert Maurer – *The Kaizen Way. One small step can change your life*

Beata Beszczyńska – *Molecular basis of stress-evoked psychiatric disturbances*

Dr Daniel G. Amen – *Unleash the Power of the Female Brain*

Phyllis A Balch – *Prescription for Nutritional Healing. A Practical A-to-Z Reference to Drug-Free Remedies Using Vitamins, Minerals, Herbs & Food Supplements*

Dr James Wilson – *Adrenal Fatigue: The 21st Century Stress Syndrome*

Dr Michael Lam – *75 Signs, Symptoms and Alerts of Adrenal Fatigue Syndrome,* https://www.drlam.com/blog/75-signs-symptoms-and-alerts-of-adrenal-fatigue-syndrome-2/1970/

Dr Lawrence Wilson – *Adrenal Burnout Syndrome,* http://www.drlwilson.com/articles/adrenal_burnout.htm

Dr Joseph Mercola – *Understanding Adrenal Function,* http://articles.mercola.com/sites/articles/archive/2000/08/27/adrenals.aspx

Stefani Ruper – *What is Pregnenolone Steal,* http://paleoforwomen.com/hpa-axis-what-is-pregnenolone-steal/

Dr. Henry Lindner – *Cortisol Deficiency,* http://hormonerestoration.com/Cortisol.html

Penny Baron – *The 10 Most Important Blood Tests* http://www.lifeextension.com/magazine/2006/5/report_blood/Page-02

Igor Mitrovic, MD – *Introduction to the Hypothalamo-Pituitary-Adrenal (HPA) Axis* http://biochemistry2.ucsf.edu/programs/ptf/mn%20links/HPA%20Axis%20Physio.pdf